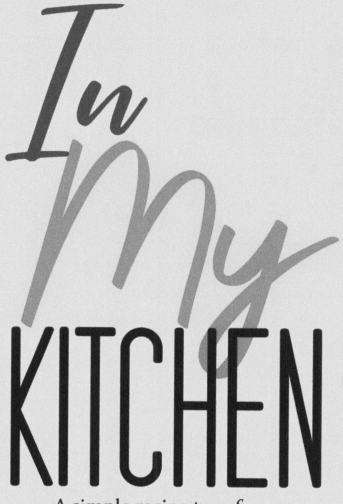

In My KITCHEN

A simple recipe tour from Africa to Minnesota

By Kasáno Mwanza
Website: www.kasanoworld.com
Instagram: @kasanoworld

Select Photos by Lucas Wells
Website: www.lucaswells.com
Instagram: @thelucaswells | @WellsFilmPhoto

Book Design by Jamacia Johnson
Website: www.amplicreative.com
Instagram: @amplicreative

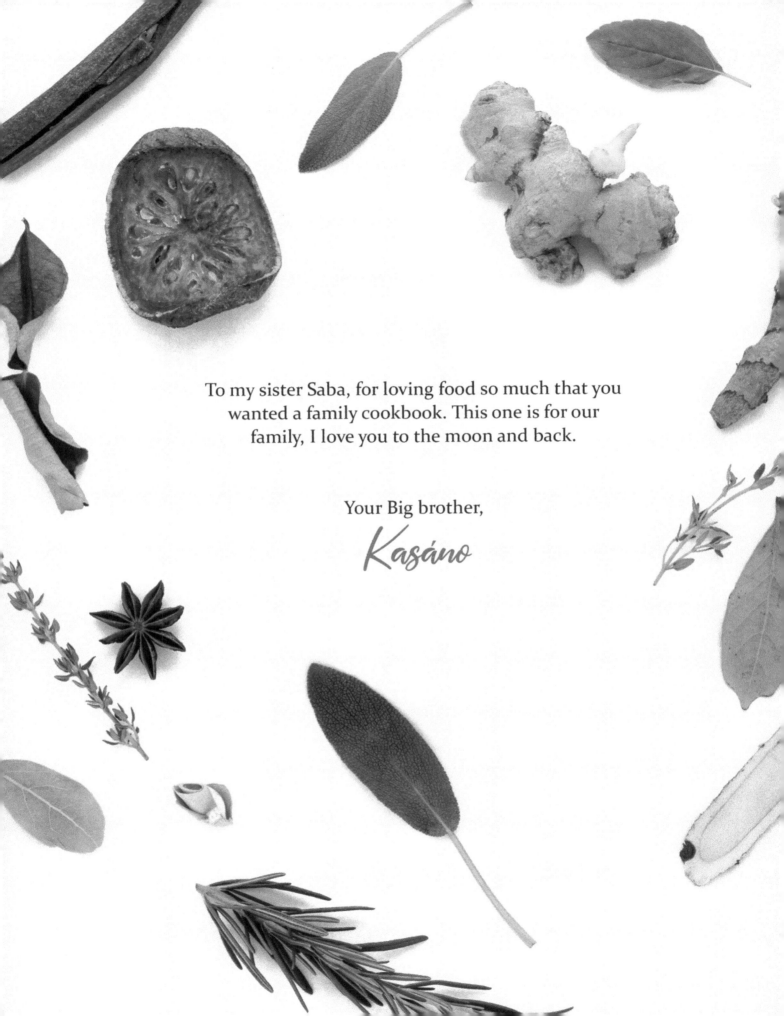

To my sister Saba, for loving food so much that you wanted a family cookbook. This one is for our family, I love you to the moon and back.

Your Big brother,

Kasáno

Contents

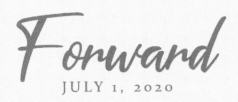

Forward

JULY 1, 2020

Breaking bread with your family, or with a group of friends, is a way to be alive together in a nourishing way. The meal brings life and regeneration to all who partake. But it is much, much more than this. By sharing the meal, we come together to celebrate the ties that bind us close. Or we can meet for the first time, and the filling flavors of the meal become the bridge that spans our difference. We can explore the past, the present, and the uncertain, imagined future. We connect through laughter and the sensual pleasure of tasting food and filling our bellies with sustenance...and love. We feed our souls and the souls of the people we care about.

My mother Jeanne, my grandmother Pearl, and my great aunt Gladdie fed me Celtic staples for decades: rye bread, the potato, the turnip, the parsnip, the cow, the pig, a turkey now and then. Though I make the fifth generation since immigrating from the Erin Isle, the Irish ways were set. The dinner table was our family moment most nights, large holiday gatherings and family reunions were annual events. The food and drink mattered. Every January 1st, my mother would cook a heavenly Pork Roast with Sauer Kraut, saying it was an Irish tradition to eat an animal that roots forward. We were a family choosing to burn the regrets of the past and focus on the sure-to-be good days to come in the new year.

When I entered the family of my wife through marriage, I sat down for meals at an entirely new table. Suddenly, I was introduced to the food of the Rio Grande Valley and Mexico; fresh corn tortillas, the tamale, the burrito; fragrant and zesty spices like cumin and cilantro; green things like jalapeno or habanero peppers and nopales (cactus); the ripe red look, smell, and taste of the tomato and the hot pepper. Cooking with my mother-in-law Maria Garcia Smith became a glorious family introduction. I learned how to make the traditional Mexican family favorites, but also came to know more about the history of my new mother. As we made the masa, the corn flour used to wrap the savory meats of the Christmas tamale, she also taught me about unconditional love and how to nourish a family.

When my wife and I were able to visit and live in Mexico, the land of her grandparents, we found ways to eat like the locals. On our second visit, we were welcomed by someone that I had only met over the phone, a friend of a friend that had agreed to help me connect with the theatre community of Mexico. This almost stranger Otto Minera arrived at the Mexico City airport first thing in the morning to shuttle us to our hotel. He introduced himself and then asked us the most important question he would ask during our entire stay: "would you like to eat breakfast at a chain restaurant like Sanborn's or at an indigenous place?" We chose indigenous, and made a friend for life.

Otto took us to what looked from the outside like an old automobile service station, with two bays that had large sheets of thick, blurry plastic masking each of the garage doors. In one bay were the old women, cooking sweet coffee in huge pots, stirring it slowly with a spoon as long as one's arm. Other women were cooking the eggs and the chorizo by a makeshift stove, or tending to the beans and rice, or grilling hot tortillas on a wood fire.

We sat down in the other bay at a long picnic table, placed end to end with three or four other tables just like it, and we enjoyed one of the best meals we had ever had. It was the beginning of a great visit, but, more importantly, the beginning of a beautiful friendship with our host Otto.

When we spent a month in Tanzania working with the Benedictine Sisters, we traveled for two full days, with only a brief stopover in Doha, Qatar. When we finally arrived at our destination, the St. Scholastica Primary School for disabled children near Bagamoyo, our host Sister Godenzia and three other nuns sang and danced to welcome us as our bus pulled into the compound. It was past 11 p.m. but we were immediately brought into the house and offered a meal. We ate meat and a maise paste called Ugali, some rice and beans, and sweets for a light desert. Though my wife Rachel and her colleague David had been Godenzia's professors back in Minnesota, the rest of the group, a dozen college students were strangers. They welcomed all of us to the dinner table like long lost relatives.

We traveled far inland to the Chipole Monastery near Songea, and again food was at the center of our welcome and new friendships with the sisters. In addition to the three meals of the day, which we took with Sister Adoratta, the Priest of the diocese, and Brother Luka, the director of the health clinic, the nuns also took tea at mid-morning and mid-afternoon. We were told that we were not to skip these breaks. The sisters knew that we, being Americans, might choose to work through these respites. The chance to gather five times a day to eat together, to share stories, and to ponder whatever was on our minds was a gift we learned always to accept.

Whenever I begin a project and gather a group that needs to work together – on a play production or a new community initiative – I start with food. Taking a meal with each other generates a sense of shared life, of a common purpose. This act acknowledges that all of us need the same things that life has to offer; food and nourishment; family and friends; a brief respite from the grind of work and or the thrill of adventure; a community that reflects our common quest to be refreshed and refueled each day. I call it the Breaking of the Bread.

Sitting down to have a meal together is the most wonderful form of fellowship. Creating a meal together, especially when it has been handed down to us by our elders and loved ones, is how community is made. It is why it endures. In short, food is love.

As you read through these recipes, or try one out with a loved one, or cook once more that meal you remember being offered by one of your ancestors, feel the love. It is baked into everything that makes cooking, eating, and gathering a crucial part of a happy and meaningful life.

Wishing you sustenance, love, peace, and good health

Bill Payne

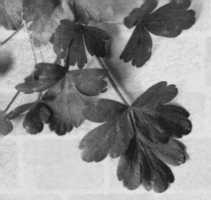

Acknowledgements

There is a strength and purpose in preservation, in collecting one of our common interests, and in generational wealth. I believe that by putting this cookbook together we attain a piece of each subject, and it is only by doing so together that this idea came to fruition. Thank you for taking the time to pull together the recipes, thank you for taking the time to find the photos, thank you for investing your time in this worthwhile idea, and thank you for letting me creatively organize one of the topics that we enjoy to the fullest. I had a great time trying some of the recipes, and I really hope they bring you as much joy as they brought me.

A huge thank you to the wonderful and talented Jamacia Johnson for the graphic design, to the talented Lucas Wells for the photography, to my multi-talented friend Alan Bach for investing his time and skillful Christmas card calligraphy, and to my dear friend the incomparable Bill Payne for writing the foreword to my family's cookbook. As Maya Angelou would say,

"I've learned that people will forget what you did, people will forget what you said, but people will never forget how you made them feel".

To Jamacia, Lucas, Alan, and Bill...Thank you for making me and my family feel special. You are a part of something we hope to keep for generations, and the gratitude you deserve is deeper than words.

To My Family

May this recipe tour from Africa to Minnesota bring us, and all In Our Kitchen, the happiest of times as we celebrate and remember each other.

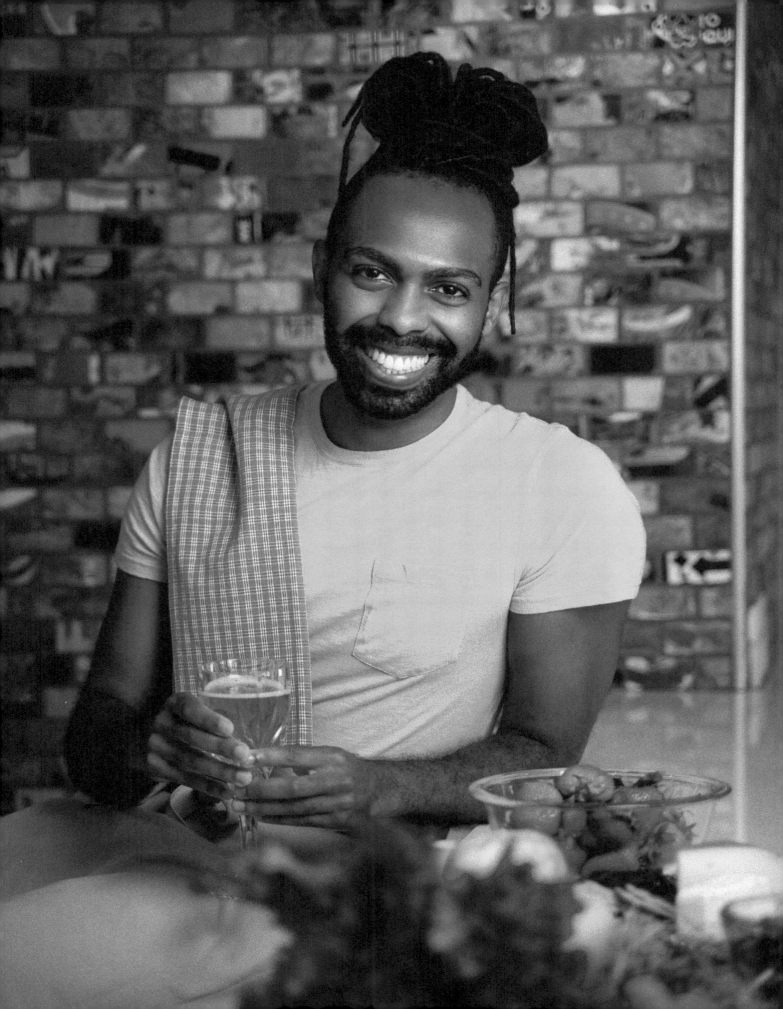

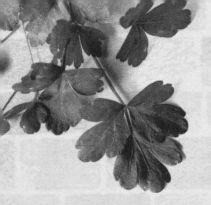

A Family Gift

A few months ago I was sitting on my couch listening to a novel (via Audible) that was set during the reign of King Louis XIV (14th) at his decadent Chateau de Versailles. It reminded me of my trips to Versailles, Italy, and the United Kingdom, but most of all it reminded me of an idea that was wildly popular for centuries. An idea that always left me impressed with its ability to remain anchored in inclusion. The fruition of this idea had the boldness to proclaim who belonged, where they came from, where they presently reside, and it even diverged subtle information about individuals if you were privy to their personal stories. It might not be as popular in the United States, or around the world due to present time, but it spoke to me.

Even through my last trip it spoke to me. Almost like a giant stop-sign, that same idea was present in London as I walked through Kensington Palace, the Harry Potter streets of Oxford, Castel de San Angelo in Rome, and the lovable Chateau de Versailles in Versailles, France. There it was…grinning at me with a hue of red that was more comforting than caution, more loving than halt, and with the request to relish instead of turning off.

There was affection and a sense of pride to its use; a bold reminder that you belonged. It was about a group who stood in solidarity, unified without hesitation, and this simple idea did nothing but belt it over and beyond the mountains. Maybe a little exaggerated, I know. The point was that it didn't matter if you were the runt of the pack, or the Hercules and/or Xenia warrior princess of the pack. You belonged.

During that very trip I decided to see the changing of the guard in London. As I stood in front of Windsor Castle I kept staring at the British Crest on the large gates, and was surprised when a tear streamed down my face. I realized I was in awe of the rich history, the lineage, and the amount of documented material that gets passed down to each new generation in their family… how this Crest symbolized this family. At the core, that's what they were/are…a family.

...And there it was again, grinning at me and asking to relish. In a sea of people in front of Windsor Castle, I stared, I cheered, and blinked through my tears.

So, back to a few months ago, I decided to stop listening to my novel, and this time I would do something about it before this feeling and idea was forgotten once again.

With it fresh in my heart and mind, I would create inclusion, I would proclaim my love to those I call family, I would share where we came from, I would honor each of our ancestors, I would be thankful for our present location and closeness, and I would create subtle passages of information for those who know us well.

I would create our family crest...one that includes us all.

A motto is common with a family crest, and so I vow the following in Latin;
- "Amare. Vivere. Ora. Cogitare. Dare."
- Love. Live. Pray. Think. Dare.
- I promise to love, even in my darkest days.
- I promise to live fully.
- I promise to pray for, and have faith in, my family and myself.
- I promise to think through my actions, and to be patient. We all have different ways of thinking and communicating.
- I promise to dare myself to take risks. If change is what I seek, I must be the catalyst.

So with my deepest love, and an overwhelming pride for this family, I present our family crest. May we collectively stand united, and may this family crest be a reminder that you, your spouse, and your kin forevermore belong.

With Love Always,

Kasáno

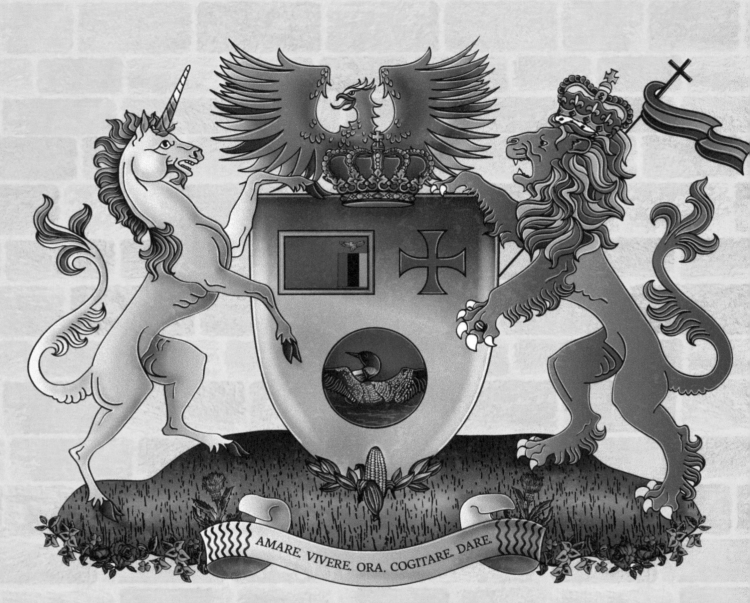

AMARE. VIVERE. ORA. COGITARE. DARE.

Family Crest Art by Alexandra Lee

Preface

MEMORY 1

It was a warm sunny day in Lusaka, Zambia, and the breeze was pleasant. We were on our shaded veranda which overlooked our back yard. Ahead of us was a mango tree, full or ripe mangos for the plucking, with branches laced with vibrant green leaves that shaded the space and sprawled upward. I was nestled on my mothers lap, and it was finally lunch time. My older brother, older sister, and the kids from next door played to their hearts content. They had already eaten, and could now play what was probably cops & robbers. My ears could faintly catch the giggles and the sound of feet hitting the ground as they ran and squealed in laughter. I was hungry and mom was feeding me shima.

Shima; A Staple food that can be described as a thicker and pliable version of porridge. Depending on what south-central region of Africa you are in, you're most likely to find a version of it. You scoop a portion with your fingers and massage it into a ball with one hand (almost like you would squeeze a stress ball). You then dip it into sauces and/or pick up anything else prepared before devouring it all in one bite. Definitely a finger-food.

My favorite part was mom would hide a piece of beef inside the shima, and would switch between just shima and the sauce and a little treasure in the shima. It made me appreciate the difference between the sauce and the beef. The sauce was thick, beef and tomato based, and left you yearning for another bite. The beef was tender enough for a toddler to chew and swallow, fresh, and dare I say it - moist. The flavor was beyond delicious, it was magnificent. This meal was lovingly cooked, it was mastery.

MEMORY 2

I believe I was seven or eight years old. We had just ascended into the air and the plane was leveling off. I remember the P.A. speaker coming on and the captain, my father, addressing the passengers. It was always exciting to hear dad talk on the speaker. He would mention that his family was aboard the flight, and we would giggle and squeal until my mother had enough. During the flight he came back to see us, and I remember him saying that once we've reached our destination we'll be able to taste the air. I thought that was odd...taste the air? Knowing me I probably eye rolled in my excitement.

We finally arrived in Bombay, India and everything was a blur until we took a step outside. The fresh air brushed and caressed my face, and whilst in appreciation my eyes closed because this air wasn't vacant. What caressed my face and brushed my sense of smell was what I can now describe as faint traces of cumin, curry, and clover. I exhaled and my taste buds began to salivate. As I took a deep breath to once more take in the scents, my mouth opened and the result made my eyes blink wide open. What I was smelling... I could taste. I was shocked and the smile plastered on my face would have proven just how amazing I thought it was. The last thing I remember thinking, while fully smiling, was that dad was totally right.

MEMORY 3

It all started when we stopped over to the big cabin to say hi. After removing our shoes and running over to grab a handful of sugary love, starbursts, she proclaimed that she ran out. Sure enough Mimi was always prepared, she had a bowl of cherries ready. I hadn't given cherries very much thought, but I said "sure, I'll try some". I loved every minute of those cherries and I'm sure my face was dramatic enough to show it. For the next few years, anytime I would come up to say hi, Mimi would have fresh cherries for me to take home. I always felt special, and the truth is that she had that kind of gift. She genuinely knew how to make you feel special, and it was in the small things she would do and say... it was in the way that she loved. It's not odd that every time I see, taste, or eat cherries...she's my first thought. She was warm, kind, and love... I miss her.

Food has power beyond nutrients, shape, color, texture, and weight. It can transport you to a small corner of your memory that lays etched in the lemon frosting of a cake. If you let it, it can help you revisit those precious moments time-and-time again in the form of a recipe. Amongst many, the one thing that binds all humans together is the need to eat. The important part of that sentence is the word together. We may come from different backgrounds, have had different experiences, the hues of our skin may lack resemblance, and our features may not curve the same way. Yet...I will always choose you. You are my family and it will be my pleasure to prove and preserve my love for us. You are the carrot cake at Christmas, the margarita to start the fun, the chocolate fudge of the century, the fish fry that bring us together, and the Ethiopian cuisine that introduces a new year. We are woven in recipes that helped shape us, and will help shape how the youngest will teach their children. They're not just recipes, they're family.

As you leaf through the pages of this cookbook, I hope you enjoy them. Each recipe has been added by a family member, and some new ones have been placed by me in order to equip and enhance. May this book preserve our memories, may it push us to discover and even learn something new, and may it be a testament to our bond in togetherness.

With Much Love Always,

Kasáno

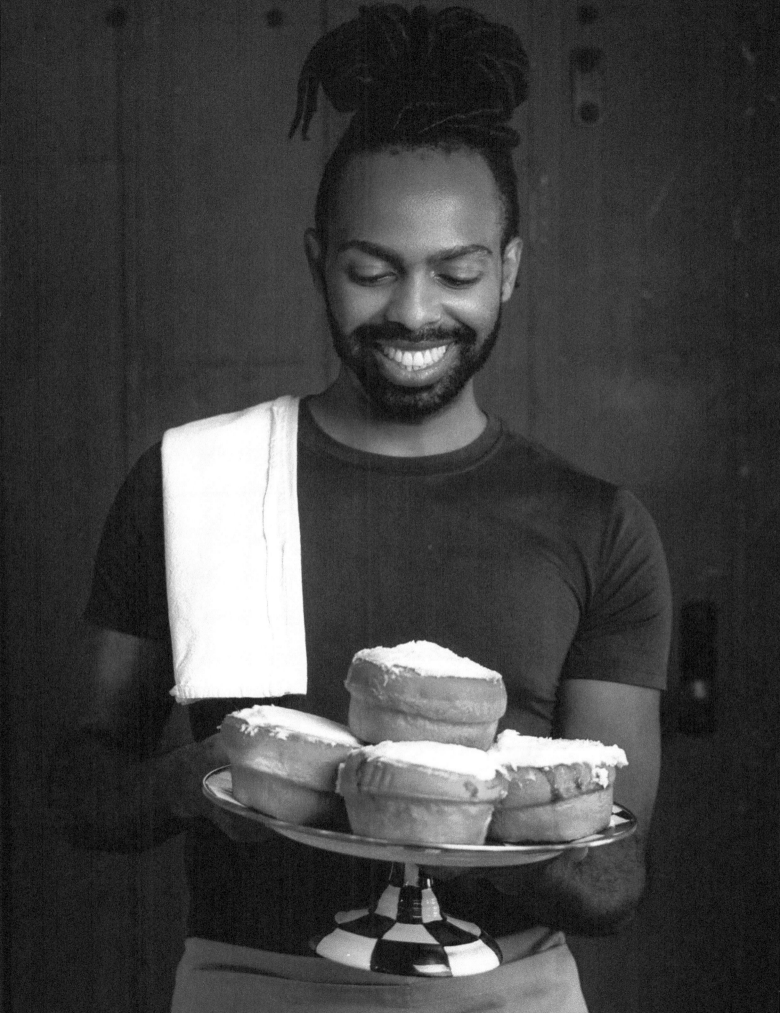

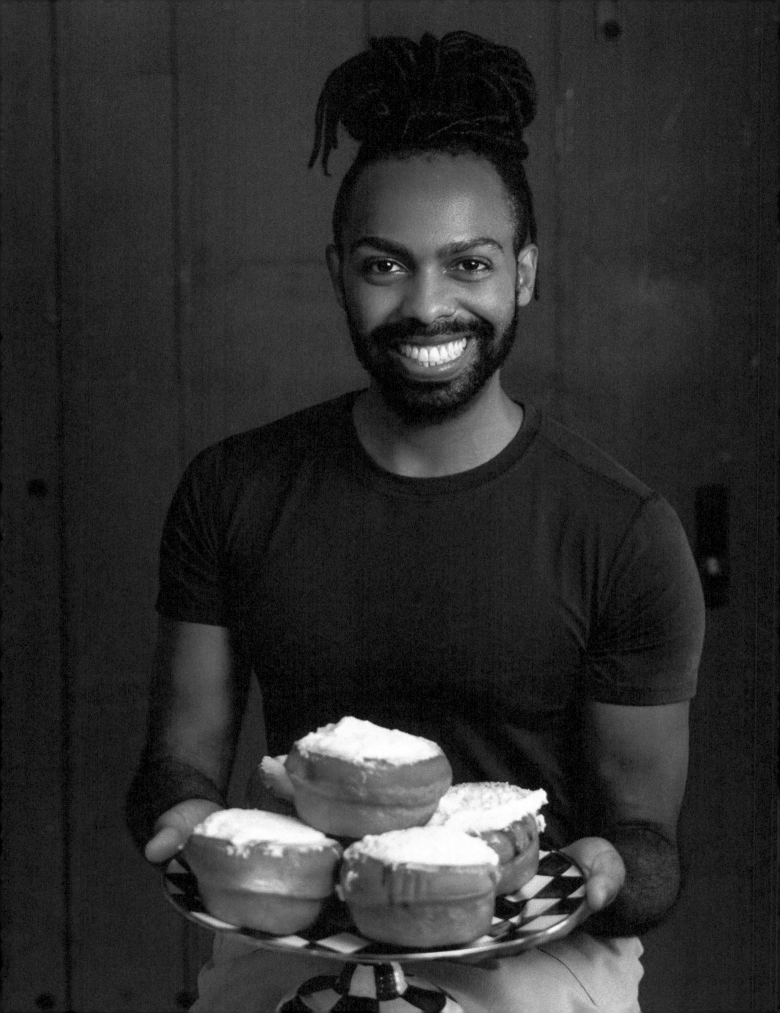

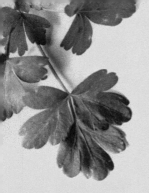
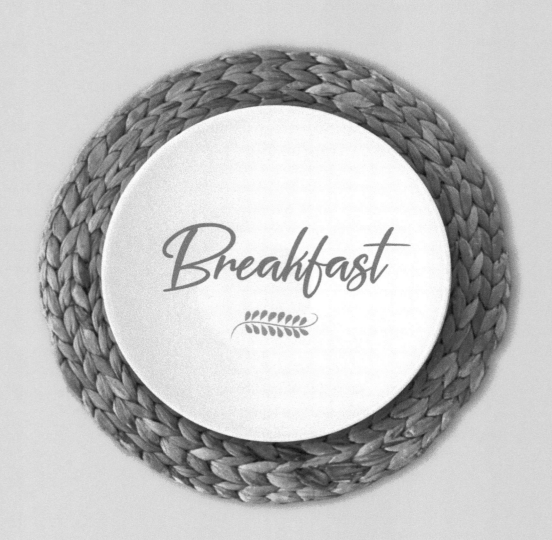
Breakfast
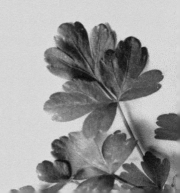

Always Avocado Toast

Makes 4 servings - 2 pieces per serving

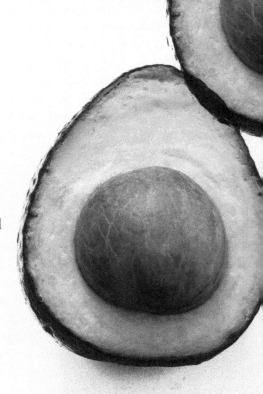

INGREDIENTS:

2 whole medium ripe avocados, skin and pit removed

2 1/2 tablespoons fresh lemon juice

1/4 teaspoon sea salt

8 slices artisan bread *(any bread)*

1 tablespoon olive oil

4 small heirloom tomatoes, sliced into 16 rounds

Hand-full of fresh basil leaves, chopped

1/3 cup sunflower sprouts

2 tablespoons chives, chopped

Salt & pepper optional

PREPARATIONS:

1. Heat the grill to medium high.
2. Place avocados in a bowl, mash with a fork, then add lemon juice and sea salt. Use plastic wrap to cover and press it down on top of avocado to prevent it from discoloring. Chill in fridge until ready to use.
3. Brush the olive oil on each side of bread slices. Place bread on grill grate. Grill until golden; flip to other side and repeat.
4. Spread approximately 2 tablespoons of avocado mixture on each piece of toast. Top that with two slices of tomato, a sprinkle of the chopped basil leaves, approximately 2 tablespoons sunflower sprouts, and a pinch of the chopped chives. Sprinkle with sea salt and pepper, if desired.

What makes this recipe for me is the basil leaves. I will literally eat anything with fresh basil leaves!

My sister Saba is a huge fan of avocado toast, so this makes me think of her. It's a slightly bougie version of avocado toast, but your taste buds will thank you! If you're in the mood for something hot, but still want this as well, try adding some hot scrambled eggs on each slice! Enjoy with a fork and knife!

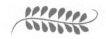

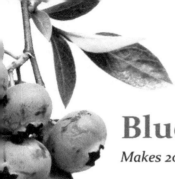

Blueberry Streusel Muffins

Makes 20 muffins

INGREDIENTS:

3 1/2 cups all purpose flour

1 1/2 cups granulated sugar

4 1/2 teaspoons baking powder

1 teaspoon baking soda

1 teaspoon kosher salt

2 cups buttermilk, shaken

1/2 teaspoon Vanilla extract

1/4 pound (1 stick) unsalted butter, melted and cooled

1 1/2 teaspoons grated lemon zest

2 extra-large eggs

2 cups fresh blueberries (2 half pints)

FOR STREUSEL TOPPING:

3/4 cup all-purpose flour

1/2 cup light brown sugar, lightly packed

1 teaspoon ground cinnamon

1/4 teaspoon kosher salt

4 tablespoons (1/2 stick) cold unsalted butter, diced

PREPARATIONS:

1. Preheat the oven to 375 degrees. Make sure to line muffin tins with paper liners.
2. Sift the flour, sugar, baking powder, baking soda, and salt into a large bowl and blend with your hands.
3. In a separate bowl, whisk buttermilk mixture and vanilla extract into the flour mixture with a fork, mixing just until blended. Fold the blueberries into the batter. Don't overmix!
4. With an ice cream scoop or large spoon, scoop the batter into the prepared cups, fill them a little over 3/4 full but not fully.

FOR TOPPING:

1. Place all ingredients in the bowl of a food processor fitted with steel blade and pulse until the butter is in very small pieces.
2. Pour into a bowl and rub with your fingers until crumbly. Spoon about 1 tablespoon of the streusel on top of each muffin. Bake the muffins for 20 to 25 minutes, until golden brown.

When I haven't seen my mother for a while I try to find a time to take her out for tea and muffins. She loves a good blueberry muffin, though we've had our fun trying different muffins with our tea around Uptown in Minneapolis. This one's for mom, its great with a cup of tea!

Breakfast Casserole

Makes 6 to 8 servings

INGREDIENTS:

2 1/2 cups herb-seasoned croutons

2 cups shredded sharp cheddar cheese (about 5 1/2 ounces)

1/4 pound sliced mushrooms (about 1 1/2 cups)

2 pounds bulk sausage

6 eggs

2 1/2 cupsmilk

1 10 3/4-ounce can cream of mushroom soup

3/4 teaspoon dry mustard

PREPARATIONS:

1. Preheat oven to 300 degrees.
2. Grease 8x8 -inch baking dish, then arrange a single layer of the croutons in the bottom of the dish. Sprinkle cheese and mushrooms evenly over croutons.
3. Cook sausage enlarge skillet, breaking into chunks, until browned, about 15 minutes. Drain thoroughly on paper towels. Place sausage over cheese and mushrooms. Beat eggs, milk, mushroom soup, and mustard in medium bowl. Pour over sausage.
4. Bake for 1 1/2 hours or until set. Serve hot.

Butterscotch-Glazed Cinnamon Rolls

Makes 18 rolls

INGREDIENTS:

10 tablespoons unsalted butter

1 cup milk

400 grams all-purpose flour, more as needed (about 3 1/2 cups)

400 grams dark brown sugar (about 2 cups)

7 grams active dry yeast (about 2 1/4 teaspoons; 1 envelope)

4 grams plus a pinch fine sea salt (about 1 teaspoon)

7 grams ground cardamom (about 3/4 teaspoon)

1 large egg

14 grams ground cinnamon (about 1 1/2 tablespoons)

2 grams freshly grated nutmeg (about 1/2 teaspoon)

1 tablespoon bourbon or apple cider

1 teaspoon vanilla extract

115 grams confectioners' sugar (about 1 cup)

PREPARATIONS:

1. In a saucepan, melt 4 tablespoons butter. Add milk and heat until just warm to the touch (120 to 130 degrees). Pour into a large bowl. In a separate bowl, whisk together flour, 100 grams or 1/2 cup brown sugar, yeast, 4 grams or 1 teaspoon salt and cardamom. Slowly beat flour mixture into butter mixture using an electric mixer set with the paddle attachment. Beat in egg, then beat until dough comes together in a ball, about 3 minutes; it should be slightly tacky but not sticky. If sticky, beat in more flour, 1 tablespoon at a time.

2. Turn dough out onto lightly floured work surface. Knead until smooth and elastic, about 2 minutes. Form into ball. Transfer to a large, lightly oiled bowl. Cover with plastic wrap and a dish towel. Let rise in a warm place until doubled in volume, 2 - 3 hours.

3. Meanwhile, in a small saucepan over medium-low heat, melt 4 tablespoons butter. Cook until the foam subsides and the butter turns a deep nut brown; cool to room temperature.

4. In a small bowl, whisk together 150 grams or 3/4 cup brown sugar, cinnamon, nutmeg and a pinch of salt.

5. Punch down dough and roll into a rectangle about 15 inches long and 12 inches wide. Using a pastry brush, coat dough with butter, leaving a 1/2-inch border all around. Sprinkle sugar mixture evenly over butter. Starting at a long end, tightly roll up dough over filling. Arrange seam side down. Cut the dough crosswise into 18 slices (about 1/2-inch thick).

6. Lightly grease two 9-inch baking pans. Transfer rolls to pan, cut side up; they will fit snugly. Cover with plastic wrap and a dish towel. Let rise in a warm place until doubled in volume, about 45 minutes.

7. Preheat oven to 375 degrees; bake rolls until golden brown, about 20 minutes. Remove from oven and cool 10 minutes. 8. See paragraph 8 under ingredients.

8. While rolls bake, place remaining 150 grams or 3/4 cup brown sugar in a small saucepan. Sprinkle with bourbon and 1/4 cup water. Bring to a simmer, stirring occasionally, and cook until sugar dissolves, about 3 minutes. Whisk in remaining 2 tablespoons butter until melted, whisk in vanilla, then turn off the heat and whisk in the confectioners' sugar. Pour warm glaze evenly over the tops of the warm rolls. Let rest for at least 20 minutes before serving to allow glaze to set.

I love this recipe, originally from Melissa Clark! I added a bit of nutmeg to give it an earthier taste closer to the cinnamon and cardamom which I love! If you don't have the ingredients for the bourbon sauce, just use Poppy's maple syrup! Delicious as well!

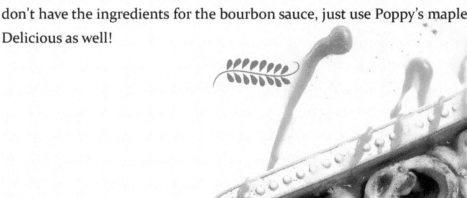

Chocolate Pancakes with Banana Flambe

PANCAKE INGREDIENTS:

4 ounces bittersweet chocolate, coarsely chopped

8 tablespoons (1 stick) unsalted butter, cut into chunks, plus 2 to 3 tablespoons unsalted butter, at room temperature.

2 large eggs

2 large egg yolks

2 tablespoons plus 2 teaspoons sugar

5 tablespoons plus all-purpose flour

PREPARATION FOR PANCAKES:

1. Melt the chocolate and the 8 tablespoons butter in the top of a double boiler or in a heatproof bowl over a saucepan of barely simmering water, stirring occasionally until smooth. Remove from heat.

2. Whisk together the egg, egg yolks, and sugar in a large bowl until well mixed. Whisk in the warm melted chocolate and butter. Sift the flour over the top and fold it in.

3. Melt 1 tablespoon utter over low heat in a large nonstick sauce pan. Drop batter by heaping tablespoons into the pan and cook for 2 minutes, then turn and cook on the other side. Transfer the pancakes to a plate. Repeat with remaining batter, adding more butter to the pan if necessary. Serve the pancakes on a platter with the bananas.

Note: The pancakes can be made in advance. Before serving, reheat in a 350 F oven until heated through.

Bananas Flambe

INGREDIENTS:

1/2 cup roasted cashews, roughly chopped

1 cinnamon stick

1/2 cup honey

1/2 cup packed brown sugar

1 vanilla bean

2 bananas, cut lengthwise in half, then cut crosswise into slices

1/4 cup dark rum

Juice of 2 limes

2 tablespoons unsalted butter, cut into pieces

PREPARATION FOR BANANA'S FLAMBE:

1. Toast the cashews and cinnamon stick in a medium sauce pan over low heat for 3 to 4 minutes,   until the cinnamon smells fragrant. Set aside to cool.

2. Combine the honey and brown sugar in a large sauce pan and cook over high heat, stirring, until the brown sugar dissolves and the mixture begins to bubble.

3. With a sharp knife, split the vanilla bean lengthwise, then use the back of the knife to scrape   out the seeds. Add the seeds, pod, bananas, and cashews and cinnamon stick and sauce for 2   to 3, until heated through.

4. Remove from heat, carefully pour in the rum, and return the to the heat; don't lean over the pan, as the rum will flame up. If the rum doesn't flame, carefully light a match and hold it at the edge of the pan; the fumes of the warmed rum should flame up immediately. The flames will extinguish after the alcohol is burned off, about 1 minute.

3. Add the lime juice and remove from the heat. Swirl in the butte until melted. Remove the cinnamon stick and vanilla pod, and serve warm.

What an experience this is for breakfast! I always love cooking this recipe with company because the flambe part is somewhat of a spectacle in its own right! There are two people in my world who are geniuses at making pancakes; my late grandfather Poppy and my dear friend Alan Bach! The truth is that I always think of you two anytime I see or cook a pancake. Alan you would slay this recipe! I added some cardamom for the Banana's Flambe to push the spice a bit more. I've also found that Wildflower honey just adds to the palette. Some honeys can be too heavy and over-power the flavor. Have someone start recording right before you start the Flambe! Great way to save the memory! Enjoy!

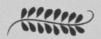

Cinnamon Rolls from Scratch

Makes 12 rolls

CINNAMON ROLLS INGREDIENTS:

1/4 cup warm water

One 1 1/4-ounce package instant yeast (2 1/4 teaspoons)

1 cup plus 1 teaspoon sugar

1 large egg, lightly beaten

1/4 cup canola oil

2 teaspoons kosher salt

1/2 cup cold water

1/2 cup boiling water

4 cups all-purpose flour, plus 1/2 cup or more as needed

2 tablespoons ground cinnamon

6 tablespoons unsalted butter, melted

FOR ICING:

1 cup confectioners' sugar

2 tablespoons milk or orange juice

PREPARATIONS:

1. For the cinnamon rolls: In the bowl of a stand mixer fitted with a dough hook, mix the warm water with the yeast and 1 teaspoon sugar. Set aside for about 5 minutes, until the mixture starts to thicken and bubble slightly. (If the mixture does not start to thicken and bubble slightly, the yeast is not working. Check the expiration date on the yeast and start over.)

2. In a large bowl, stir together 1/2 cup sugar, the egg, oil and salt. Mix in the cold water and then the boiling water. Add this to the yeast mixture and stir until well blended. With the machine on low speed, slowly add in 4 cups of flour until incorporated.

3. Knead in the mixer on low speed for about 5 minutes until smooth, adding in the extra 1/2 cup flour or more as needed so the dough isn't too sticky. Put the dough into a clean large bowl. Cover with plastic wrap and refrigerate until doubled in size, about 3 hours.

4. Meanwhile, combine the remaining 1/2 cup sugar with the cinnamon in a small bowl. Grease a 9-by-13-inch baking dish with about 1 tablespoon of the melted butter using a pastry brush.

5. Punch down the dough and place it on a lightly floured surface. Using a rolling pin, roll it into a rectangle about 20 by 10 inches, with the long edge facing you. Using the pastry brush, spread 1/4 cup of the melted butter over the top of the dough. Sprinkle the cinnamon-sugar mixture evenly over the dough. Roll up the dough, starting with the long edge facing you, into a tight cylinder. Gently squeeze the cylinder to seal it. Use a sharp knife to cut the dough into 12 even rounds. Place the rounds, cut-side down, into the prepared baking dish. There will be some space in between the rounds. Brush the tops of the rolls with the remaining 1 tablespoon melted butter. Cover the dish tightly with plastic wrap and allow the dough to rise in a warm place for 1 1/2 to 2 hours.
6. Preheat the oven to 350 degrees F. Bake the rolls until golden, 40 to 45 minutes.
7. For the icing: Meanwhile, mix the confectioners' sugar with the milk in a small bowl. When the rolls come out of the oven, drizzle the icing over the hot rolls. Serve while warm.

COOK'S NOTE

Using an electric mixer, mix the butter and the cream cheese first in large bowl until it's creamy. Once creamy, add the rest of the ingredients, but slowly add the confectioners' sugar and salt last. Should be fluffy and creamy when done.

These will win you smiles! You might also get some pleasurable grunts from how delicious each bite is, and even more for the finger-licking icing! I like my cinnamon rolls warm, which makes the frosting warm and delicious! Here's a little secret... If you can't sleep and your next day isn't busy...this is literally love on plate! A cup of honey-lavender tea by Tazo to relax you as well, its caffeine free and delicious.

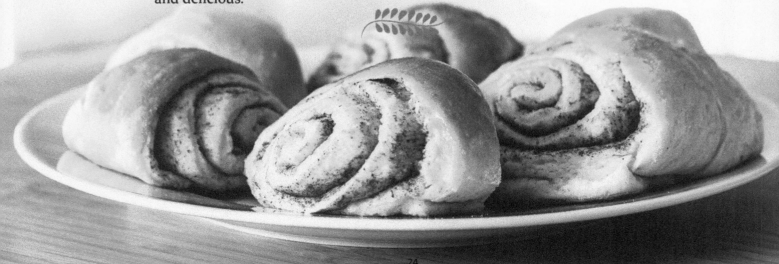

Country French Omelet

Makes 2 servings

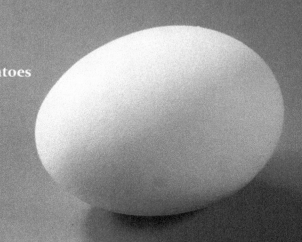

1 tablespoon good olive oil

3 slices this-cut bacon, cut into 1-inch pieces

1 cup (1-inch-diced) unpeeled Yukon Gold potatoes

1/2 teaspoon salt

1/4 teaspoon freshly ground black pepper

5 extra-large eggs

3 tablespoons 2% milk

1 tablespoon unsalted butter

1 tablespoon fresh chopped chives

1/8 teaspoon dill weed

PREPARATIONS:

1. Preheat the oven to 350 degrees.

2. Heat olive oil in a 10-inch ovenproof omelet pan over medium heat. Add the bacon and cook for 3 to 5 minutes over medium-low heat, stirring occasionally, until the bacon is browned but not crisp. Take the bacon out of the pan with a slotted spoon and set aside on a plate.

3. Place the potatoes in the pan and sprinkle with salt and pepper. Continue to cook over medium-low heat for 8 to 10 minutes, until very tender and browned, tossing occasionally to brown evenly. Remove with a slotted spoon to the same plate with bacon.

4. Meanwhile, in a medium bowl, beat the eggs, milk, 1/2 teaspoon salt, 1/8 teaspoon dill weed, and 1/4 teaspoon pepper together with a fork. After the potatoes are removed, pour the fat out of the pan and discard. Add the butter, lower the heat to low, and pour the eggs into the hot pan. Sprinkle the bacon, potatoes, and chives evenly over the top and place the pan in the oven for about 8 minutes, just until the eggs set. Slide onto a plate, divide in half, and serve hot.

Creamy Quinoa Porridge

Makes 6 servings

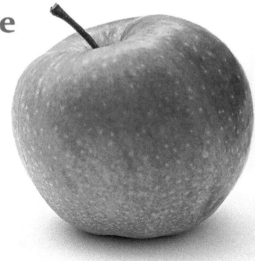

INGREDIENTS:

1/2 cup quinoa, rinsed

1 1/ 2cups chopped apple with skin *(approx.1 apple)*

1/4 cup raisins

1 teaspoon vanilla extract

1/4 teaspoon ground cinnamon

1/8 cardamom, powder

2 cups water

1/2 cup whole milk

1 1/2 tablespoons ground flaxseed

(Raw chopped walnuts, unshelled sunflower seeds, or pepitas optional)

PREPARATIONS:

1. Rinse quinoa under cold running water using a fine mesh strainer for about 30 seconds.
2. Combine quinoa, chopped apple, raisins, vanilla and cinnamon with water in a pot and bring to a boil. Reduce heat to low; cover and simmer for 20 minutes.
3. Stir in whole milk and remove from heat.
4. Spoon into bowls and top with flaxseed (1/2 tablespoon of flax seed per serving). Add raw chopped walnuts, unshelled sunflower seeds, or pepitas if desired

Want a warm breakfast, but trying to stay healthy? This is a delicious and reasonably healthy option! There's something about a warm porridge in a bowl, and taking your time to savor. There's a calmness about it! I love this recipe, originally from my cousin Justin and his wife Autumn! Best in the fall or winter, but still good all year around!

Ethiopian Spice Tea

INGREDIENTS:

1 teaspoon ground cardamom

1/2 teaspoon ground cinnamon

1/8 teaspoon ground nutmeg

1/8 teaspoon ground cloves

1 - 1 1/2 cups of water

1 Slice fresh ginger root *(about 1/4-inch-thick,)*

Wildflower honey *(for sweetness)*

PREPARATIONS:

1. Stir all ground spices together in a small bowl.
2. Bring water to a boil.
3. Add 1/8 teaspoon spice mixture and ginger and simmer 4 minutes.
4. Pour tea through a fine sieve (optional to line sieve with coffee filter) in a cup. Add honey if you want it sweetened.

This tea holds a special place in my heart and always will. My mother used to make this for us when we were kids, and still does when we visit. There's a sense of warmth that the ginger brings, and the cardamom hugs you. I would say this is best in the fall and winter time, but the truth is that this tea will always bring some sense of comfort. I usually add wildflower honey to my cup for some sweetness, I think sugar takes the tea in the wrong direction. This tea does wonders when you want to catch up with someone, want to stare at a view, a piece of art, relax on a couch with a blanket, or just need something delicious to sip while you ponder.

7152 French Toast

Makes 5-6 servings

INGREDIENTS:

1 Large Soft French Baguette

7 Eggs

2 tsp Vanilla Extract

1 tbsp Cinnamon

1 tbsp French's Yellow Mustard

Powdered Sugar

PREPARATIONS:

1. Slice baguette into 1/2" thick discs.
2. Mix remaining ingredients in small baking pan and stir till mixture is consistent.
3. Place baguette discs in pan with mixture, flip so both sides are covered in mixture.
4. Put a generous chunk of butter into a pan and put on medium heat.
5. Fill the pan with bread, cook both sides until its a beautiful golden brown.
6. Add syrup (Look at Poppy's Maple syrup recipe)
7. Lightly dust with powder sugar & enjoy with a cup of tea/coffee!

I got this recipe from my cousin Ben, and it is delicious! I think Poppy's maple syrup just takes it up a notch! Ben's little girls are huge fans of this recipe, so I thought it would be a great one to share for those who have little ones that want to help. Its a win-win for kids and also for any adults that love a good fresh toast breakfast.

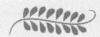

Poppy's Pancakes & Maple Syrup

INGREDIENTS:
Your favorite Pancake Mix
Oil
Eggs
Milk

PREPARATION FOR PANCAKES:
1. Mix the batter according to the directions found on the Hungry Jack box. Then add the following to the batter:
    - 2 teaspoons oil
    - 1 extra egg
2. Mix to desired consistency by increasing or decreasing the powder mixture to the batter. Thin is good for stacks of pain pancakes. Thick is good when adding blueberries to the batter.

MAPLE SYRUP INGREDIENTS:
1 cup water
2 cups brown sugar
1/2 tsp mapleine

PREPARATION FOR MAPLE SYRUP:
1. Boil the sugar and water, then add mapleine.

Many years ago, on a pontoon with a griddle, my grandpa Poppy would make these pancakes for us. My aunt and mom would bring the all the extras (scrambled eggs, ham, sausage, orange juice, etc) in a cooler. The eggs would be still be warm! We would drive the pontoon to a spot that had the biggest willow tree I can remember seeing as a kid, and Poppy would have me or my brother drop the anchor in front of the willow tree. We'd get all set up and he would pass those pancakes over, and some had blueberries! There was something magical about it. It was a warm summer day, the lake was still calm, the willow tree would would wisp with small tufts of wind, and we giggled, laughed, and enjoyed family and good food. It a memory I always think of when I see willow trees and blue berry pancakes. It's most likely the reason why my favorite tree is the willow tree.

Sunrise Smoothies

Makes 2 servings

INGREDIENTS:

1 cup chopped strawberries (5 strawberries)

1 cup chopped watermelon, seeded

1 cup chopped fresh peach

1 cup (1/2 pint)raspberry sorbet

1/4 cup freshly squeezed orange juice

Watermelon or strawberry spears (for garnish)

PREPARATIONS:

1. Place the strawberries, watermelon, peach, sorbet, and orange juice in a blender and puree until smooth and creamy. Add more orange juice if you'd like it less thick. Serve immediately in glasses with watermelon or strawberry spears.

You can also put different fruit on skewers, kebab style, and use that to stir your individual glass. That way you have a mini meal/full snack. Great if you're trying to be better about eating more fruit, or just want to add this to your breakfast!

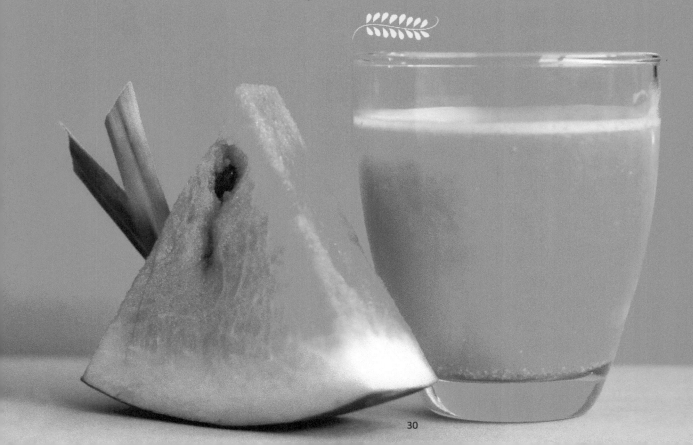

Sweet Potato-Coconut Turnovers

Makes 12 Turnovers

INGREDIENTS:

2 medium sweet potatoes, peeled

3 to 4 cups all purpose flour

1/2 cup sugar

1/2 teaspoon salt

Coconut filling (recipe follows)

8 tablespoons (1stick) unsalted butter, or as needed, divided

1 cup sour cream

2 tablespoons confectioners' sugar

Juice of 1 lime

COCONUT FILLING INGREDIENTS:

1 cup thawed frozen grated coconut or sweetened shredded coconut

1/2 cup packed dark brown sugar

1/2 cup chopped toasted cashews

1/2 cup golden raisins

2 tablespoons sesame seeds, toasted

PREPARATIONS FOR SWEET POTATO TURNOVERS:

1. To make the dough, cook the sweet potatoes in a saucepan of boiling water until tender. Drain, then press through potato ricer into a large bowl. Stir in 3 cups flour, the sugar, and salt,   mixing well, then turn out on a floured work surface and knead, adding as much of the   remaining cup of flour as necessary to achieve a smooth, workable dough. Wrap in plastic and set aside to rest for at least 30 minutes.

2. Divide the dough into 12 equal pieces, and roll each piece into a ball. One at a time, on the lightly floured surface, roll each piece into a 6-inch circle. Place 1 1/2 tablespoons of filling in the center, use your fingertips to brush a little water around the outer edge of the circle, and then carefully fold the dough in half. Crimp the edges with your fingers or a fork to seal.

3. Melt 2 tablespoons of the butter on a griddle or in a skillet over medium heat. Add 2 or 3 turnovers and fry until golden on the bottom, about 3 minutes. Turn and fry the other side,   then transfer to paper towels to drain. Fry the remaining turnovers, adding more butter as   needed. Let cool.
4. Place the sour cream in a small bowl and whisk in the confectioners' sugar and lime juice. Place dollop of the sour cream mixture on each turnover before serving.

PREPARATIONS FOR COCONUT FILLING:

1. Combine all the ingredients in a medium bowl and mix until well combined.

Sweet potatoes always remind me of Zambia, and enjoying them with family. There are so many reasons to eat sweet potatoes, and I will always find a way to put them on the table. This recipe was originally from the magnificent Marcus Samuelsson, I added a little bit of vanilla extract to warm the flavor of the sweet potato. A great way to enjoy sweet potato, and to share with company.

Uncle Jim's Sluggo Pie

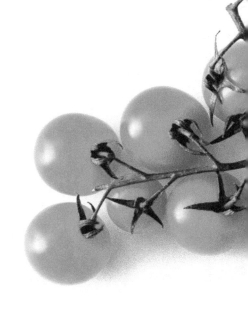

INGREDIENTS:

6x10 baking dish

Small tomato, chopped into 1/2-inch pieces

4 1/2 oz. can sliced mushrooms

1/2 large diced green pepper

Small diced ham or bacon

4 eggs

2-3 oz. 2% Milk

1/4 - 1/2 aged sharp cheddar cheese, or favorite cheese

1/4 - 1/2 cup loosely packed, coarsely chopped fresh basil leaves

PREPARATION:

1. In baking dish, combine tomato, green pepper, onion, and ham or bacon.
2. In a bowl, blend together eggs, milk, and cheese. Pour mixture into baking dish.
3. Season with salt and pepper. Tabasco is optional if you want a punch!
4. Bake for 45-50 minutes until center is firm and edges are browned.

Originally this recipe didn't have basil in it, but I tried it once and never went back! My grandpa Poppy is also Uncle Jim, and this is his recipe. Its great if you have company and want something that will feed a number of people. It's also a good one to pack in to-go containers, but because there's tomato is this one I would say its good for 2 days of to-go. Delicious for breakfast, and also for a quick lunch on the go!

Veggie, Bacon, & Quinoa Quiche Wedges

Makes 6 wedges

INGREDIENTS:

Use nonstick cooking spray

1/2 cup quinoa, rinsed and drained

1 tablespoon olive oil

2 cups sliced fresh mushrooms

1/2 cup sliced leek

1/2 cup loosely packed, coarsely chopped fresh spinach leaves

1/2 cup loosely packed, coarsely chopped fresh basil leaves

4 slices bacon, crisp-cooked and coarsely crumbled

4 eggs, lightly beaten

1 1/2 cups fat-free milk

2 oz. Gruyere or favorite cheese, freshly shredded (1/2 cup)

1/4 teaspoon salt

1/8 teaspoon black pepper

PREPARATIONS:

1. Preheat the oven to 350 degrees and coat a 9-inch pie plate with nonstick cooking spray. Spread uncooked quinoa in prepared pie plate.
2. In a 10-inch skillet heat oil over medium. Add mushrooms and leek; cook 3 to 5 minutes or just until tender, stirring occasionally. Remove from heat. Stir in spinach and bacon.
3. Spread mushroom mixture over quinoa. In a medium bowl combine remaining ingredients. Pour over mixture in pie plate (dish will be full).
4. Bake 45 to 50 minutes or until center is set and top is golden. Let stand 10 minutes before serving. Cut into wedges.

This is great if you're someone who's on the go in the morning, but you want to have something that's warm and reasonably healthy. I usually separate the wedges into to-go containers and have some fruit ready to go as well. You can also do the opposite and make this a meal at the table. A toasted (and buttered) slice of thick country bread with a fresh arugula salad (light vinaigrette) all on one plate. A cup of tea, or coffee, to round it all out. Enjoy the flavors! Its the basil that does it for me, I love it!

Recipe Notes

Recipe Notes

"The family is a community of love where each of us learns to relate to others and to the world around us."

- Pope Francis

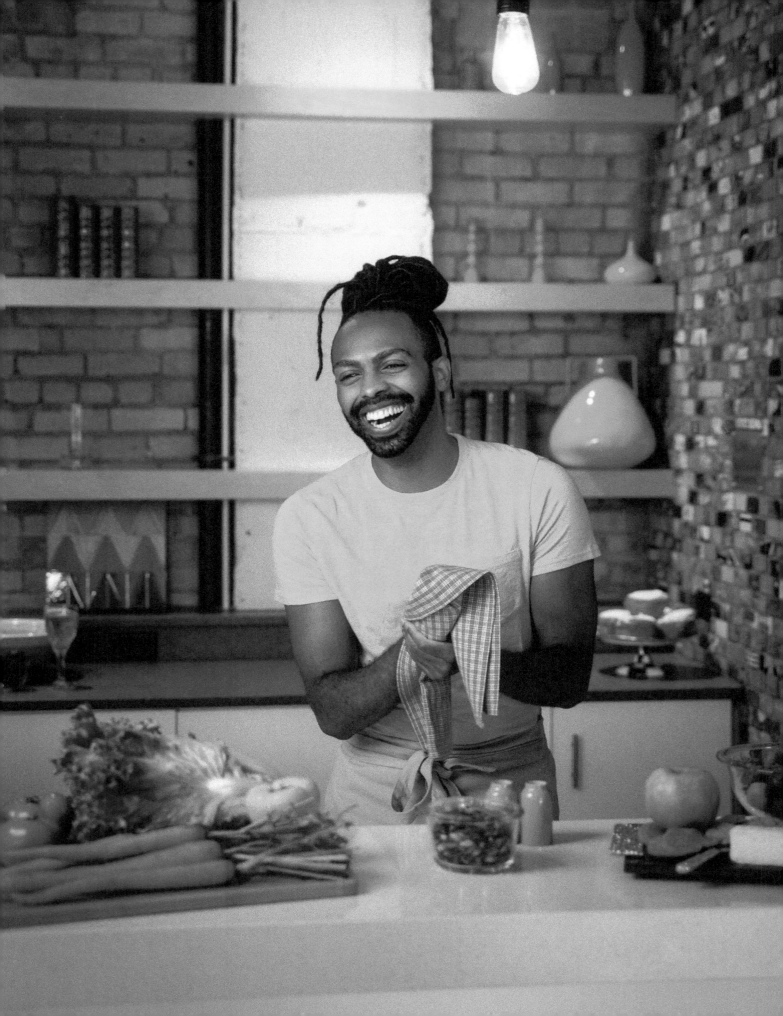

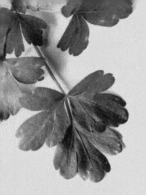
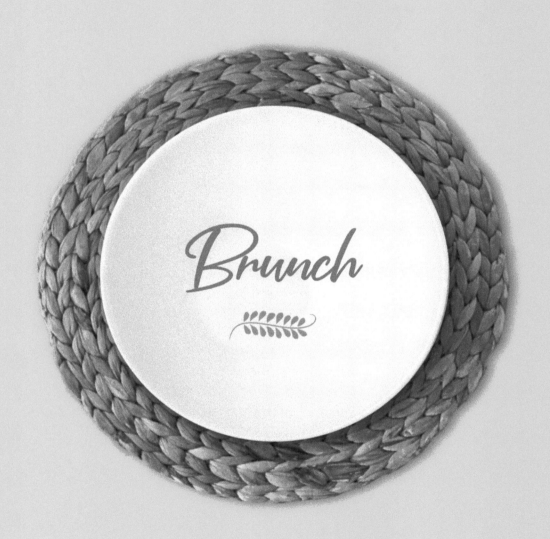

Brunch

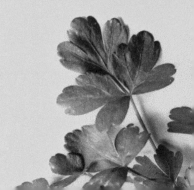

Brunch Pizza Omelet

Makes 2 HUGE servings

INGREDIENTS:

1/2 lb sweet sausage

Olive oil for pan

1 green pepper, coarsely chopped

1 large onion, coarsely chopped

1/2 pound mushrooms, coarsely chopped

1 large tomato, cut in eighths

1 tablespoon fresh basil (1 tsp. dried)

6 eggs

2 tablespoons milk

Salt & pepper to taste

Sprinkle of Parsley

1/2 teaspoon of rosemary

1/4 lb each grated Swiss and sharp cheddar cheese

1 teaspoon chives

1/2 cup dairy sour cream

PREPARATIONS:

1. Brown sausage in heavy pan, breaking into 1-inch chunks. Remove and drain on paper towels. Wipe pan with paper towels.

2. In pan: add one tablespoon olive oil, heat. Add green pepper, onion, rosemary, and mushrooms. Sauté until onions and peppers are tender, around 2-3 minutes. Remove from skillet and set aside.

3. Cut tomato into eighths and sprinkle with basil. Beat eggs with milk, salt

4. Wipe pan with paper towel. Coat pan with olive oil. When very hot (almost smoking) pour in eggs. Cook, scraping down sides to cook all liquid. When omelet begins to set, top with green peppers, onions and mushrooms. Sprinkle with parsley. Add grated cheese and let melt for 2 minutes.

5. Turn oven to broil. Top omelet with meat, the sour cream and chives. Lay tomatoes across the top. Broil until slightly brown, about 2 minutes.

Buttermilk Cheddar Biscuits

Makes 8 biscuits

INGREDIENTS:

2 cups all purpose flour

1 tablespoon baking powder

1 1/2 teaspoons kosher salt

1/2 teaspoon garlic powder

12 tablespoons (1 1/2 sticks) cold unsalted butter, diced

1/2 cup cold buttermilk, shaken

1 cold extra-large egg

1 cup grated extra-sharp Cheddar

1 egg beaten with 1 tablespoon milk

PREPARATIONS:

1. Preheat the oven to 425 degrees.

2. Place flour, baking powder, and salt in the bowl of an electric mixer fitted with the paddle attachment. With the mixer on low, add the butter and mix until the butter is the size of peas.

3. Combine the buttermilk and egg in a small glass measuring cup and beat lightly with a fork. With the mixer still on low, quickly add the buttermilk mixture to the flour mixture and mix only until moistened. In a small bowl, mix the Cheddar with a small handful of flour and garlic , with the mixer still on low, add the cheese and garlic mix to the dough. Mix only until roughly combined.

4. Dump out onto a well-floured board and knead lightly about six times. Roll the dough out to a rectangle 5 x 10 inches. With a sharp, floured knife, cut the dough lengthwise in half and then across in quarters, making 8 rough rectangles.

5. Transfer to a baking sheet lined with parchment paper. Brush the tops with the egg wash, sprinkle with sea salt, and bake for 20 to 25 minutes, until the tops are browned and the biscuits are cooked through. Serve hot or warm.

I love a good cheddar biscuit! I might need to take a lactose pill, but SO WORTH IT! I added a little garlic to this one because I think it gives a nice dimension to the cheese. Not my fault if you have more than one!

Overnight Cheese & Sausage Brunch

INGREDIENTS:

6 eggs

2 cups of milk

1 teaspoon salt

1/2 teaspoon garlic powder

1 teaspoon dry mustard

6 slices of thick french bread, cubed

1 lb ground pork sausage, *(browned, drained, and cooled)*

1 1/2 cups shredded cheddar or American Cheese

PREPARATIONS:

1. Butter a 7 x 11 or 9 x 13 pan.
2. Blend eggs, milk, salt, garlic powder, and dry mustard.
3. Put the cubed bread at the bottom of the pan, push down on the bread. Spread the ground pork sausage and cheese on top, then pour the mixture over all or it.
4. Refrigerate overnight.
5. Bake at 325 degrees uncovered.

*If you're in the Minnesota area, my cousin Ben recommends the Mexican Style Bacon from Lantto's Store in French Lake, MN. He says "trust me, it's the best you've ever had!"

Sausage Gravy Brunch

Makes 5 cups

INGREDIENTS:

1 1/2 pounds bulk pork sausage

1 cup onion, chopped

1/4 cup Gluten free flour mix (or regular flour)

3 cups milk

2 teaspoons fresh thyme

1/2 teaspoon garlic powder

Salt & Pepper

PREPARATIONS:

1. In 12-inch skillet cook pork sausage, chopped onion, and garlic powder on medium-high until meat is browned and onion is tender. Do not drain.

2. Sprinkle with1/4 cup Gluten Free Flour mix; whisk into meat mixture.

3. Gradually add 3 cups of milk, whisking constantly. Cook and stir until thickened and bubbly. Cook and stir 1 minute more. Season to taste with salt and black pepper.

4. Stir in 2 teaspoons chopped fresh thyme.

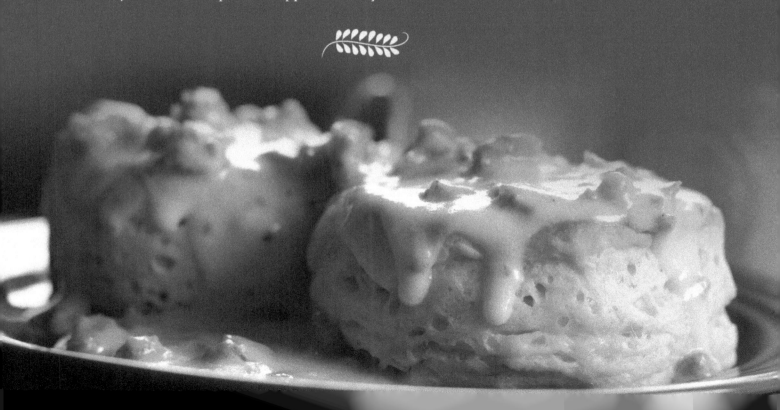

Shrimp Grits

Makes 4 servings

INGREDIENTS:

2 pounds large, head-on, tail-on shrimp (31/35 count, but can 20/25 count)

6 cups water

1 tablespoon kosher salt

2 to 3 bay leaves

1 cup stone-ground grits

1 tablespoon unsalted butter

1 tablespoon fresh lemon juice

2 teaspoons hot sauce

1 teaspoon Old Bay Seasoning

4 thin slices of bacon (rashers)

4 scallions, finely chopped

Small clove of garlic, chopped (1/2 teaspoon)

PREPARATIONS:

1. Remove the heads and tails from the shrimp and save for making shrimp broth. Devein the shrimp and refrigerate while making the shrimp broth. Rinse the shrimp shells with cool water.

2. Heat a 4-quart pot over medium- high heat. Add the shrimp shells and cook until pink. Cover with the water and bring to a boil. Reduce the heat to a simmer and continue to cook, uncovered, for 45 minutes to an hour (looking for this to reduce to quart). Strain the broth and cool over an ice bath.

3. Combine the cooled broth with the salt and bay leaves, whisking until the salt is dissolved. Set the grits in a 4-quart pot and top with the shrimp. Cover the grits and shrimp with the brine and stash in the fridge for at least 6 hours or overnight.

4. After the 6-hour brine: Remove any chaffs or hulls from the grits that may be floating on the surface. Remove the shrimp from the brine.

5. Bring the grits to a simmer over medium-high heat, whisking continuously until the grits boil, to avoid lumps. Reduce the heat and cook the grits for 30 to 35 minutes, until tender and creamy. Add the butter and stir to combine. Cover to keep warm while cooking the shrimp.

6. Toss the shrimp with the lemon juice, hot sauce and Old Bay seasoning. Set aside.

7. Cook the bacon in a large cast-iron skillet over medium-high heat until crisp. Remove from the pan to paper towels to drain. Add the shrimp and cook until pink, two minutes per side. Coarsely chop the bacon, return it to the pan, and add the scallions and garlic. Stir to combine and sauté. About 3 minutes

8. To serve, ladle the grits into a bowl and scatter the shrimp and bacon mixture over.

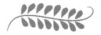

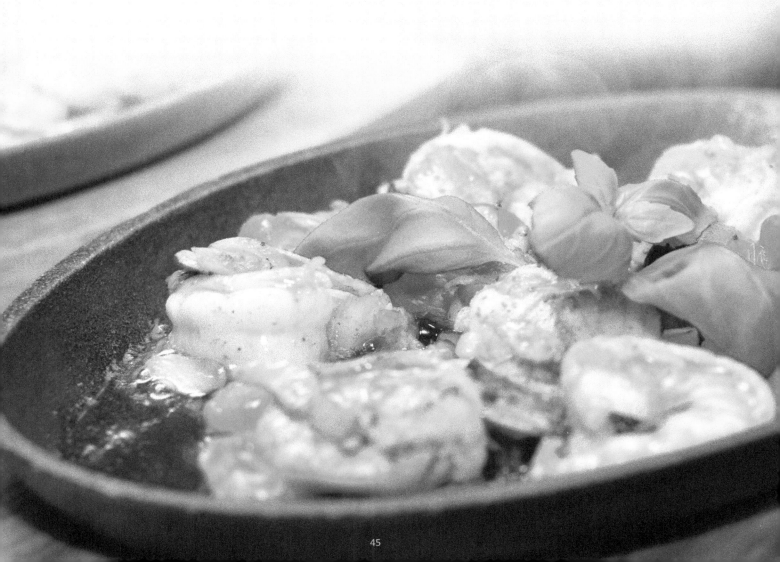

Steak & Egg Tacos with Ranchero Sauce

Makes 4 servings

INGREDIENTS FOR RANCHERO:

3/4 cup canned diced tomatoes with juice

2 to 3 teaspoons minced jalapeño or Serrano Chile, without seeds, to taste

1 small clove of garlic, minced (About 1 teaspoon)

1 teaspoon chili powder

1/2 teaspoon ground cumin

1/4 teaspoon dried oregano

1/4 teaspoon paprika

Pinch of kosher salt, for taste

2 tablespoons chopped fresh cilantro

1/2 cup chicken broth

INGREDIENTS FOR THE TACOS:

8 (5 to 6 inch) corn tortillas

1 teaspoon ground cumin

1/2 teaspoon sweet or hot paprika

1/2 teaspoon kosher salt, plus more to taste for eggs

1 (12-ounce) New York strip or sirloin steak, about 1 inch thick

1 1/2 teaspoons plus 2 tablespoons butter, softened, divided

6 eggs

Ground pepper, to taste

3/4 cup (3 ounces) shredded Monterey Jack cheese

1/4 cup chopped green onions

1/2 ripe avocado, sliced

1/4 cup loosely packed cilantro sprigs

PREPARATIONS:

1. For the Ranchero sauce: Combine all the sauce ingredients in a small sauce pan, and bring to a simmer over medium heat. Add a generous pinch of salt, and adjust the heat to maintain a gentle simmer. Cook until sauce slightly thickens and the tomatoes soften, 20 minutes. Puree the sauce in a blender (or with an immersion blender) until smooth. Add the cilantro, and taste for salt. Set aside in a warm spot.

2. For the tacos: Preheat the oven to 350 degrees. Stack the tortillas in 2 stacks of 4 each, wrap each stack in foil and set aside.

3. Combine the cumin, paprika and 1/2 teaspoon kosher saltine's a small dish. Sprinkle all over the steak.

4. Heat a heavy skillet (preferably well-seasoned cast iron) over medium-high heat. When the skillet is very hot, sear the steak (with no added fat) until well browned, about 2 minutes. Flip the steak, and immediately transfer to the oven. Place the packets of tortillas in the oven at the same time. After 6 minutes, check the steak for doneness either with an instant-read thermometer or by making small cut with a pairing knife. Cook until the internal temperature is 125 degrees for medium rare or 130 degrees for medium. Transfer the steak to a cutting board to rest , and spread a small pat (1 1/2 teaspoons) of butter over the surface. Turn off the oven, but leave the tortillas inside to keep them warm while you cook the eggs.

5. Whisk the eggs in a bowl, and season with salt and pepper to taste. Melt the remaining 2 tablespoons of butter in a medium nonstick skillet over medium heat. Add the eggs and cook, stirring gently with a heat-proof rubber spatula to form large curds. When the eggs are soft and fluffy, stir in the cheese and green onions, and remove from the heat.

6. Carve the steak across the grain into thin slices. Pull the tortillas from the oven, and open the packets carefully, avoiding the steam. Fill each tortilla with scrambled eggs, and then add steak, avocado, and ranchero sauce. Garnish with cilantro. Serve immediately, passing any extra sauce at the table.

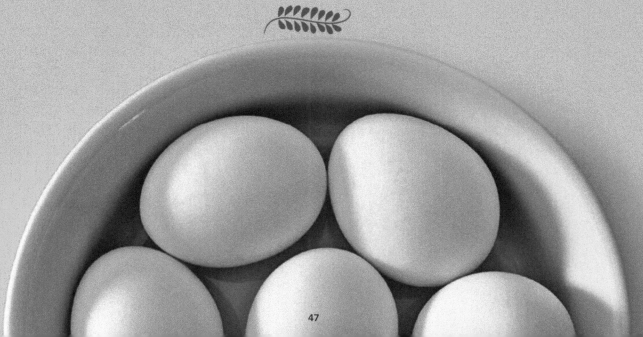

Recipe Notes

Recipe Notes

"

"I have dream that my four little children will one day live in a nation where they will not be judged by the color of their skin, but by the content of their character."

- Martin Luther King

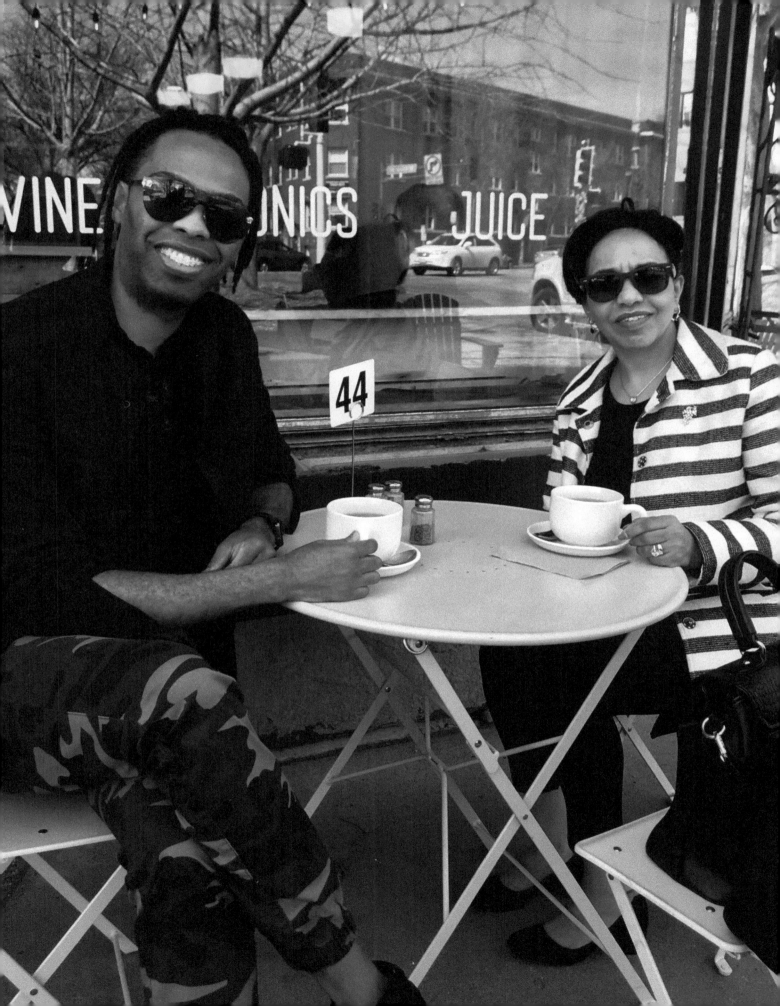

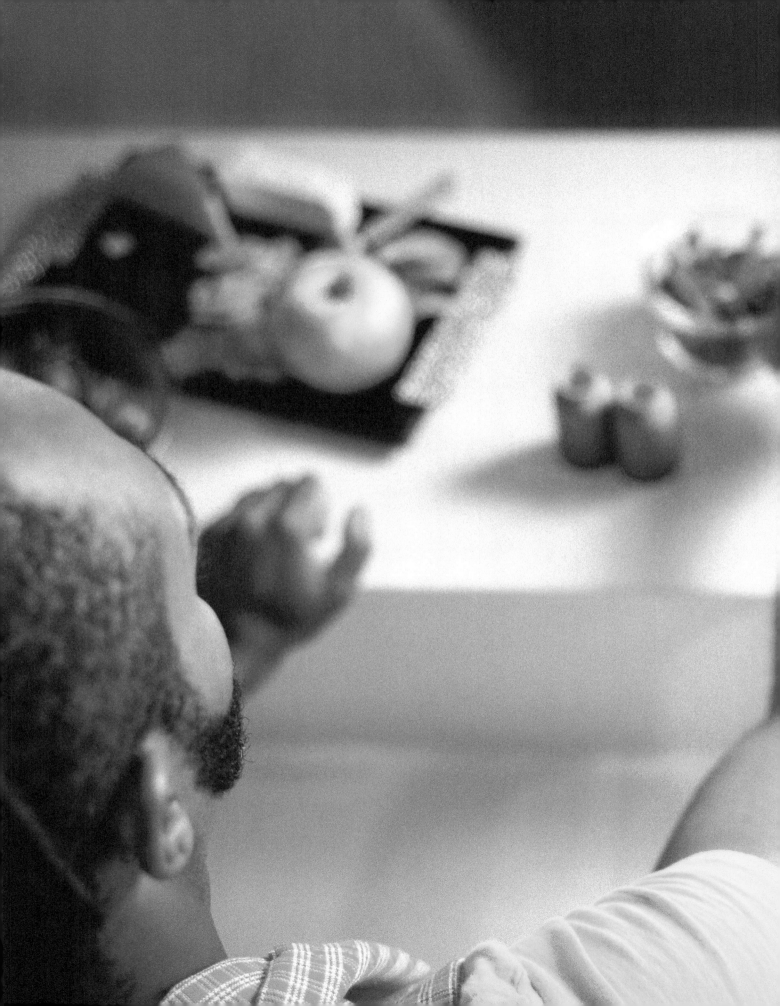

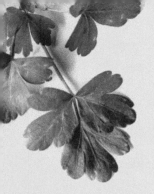
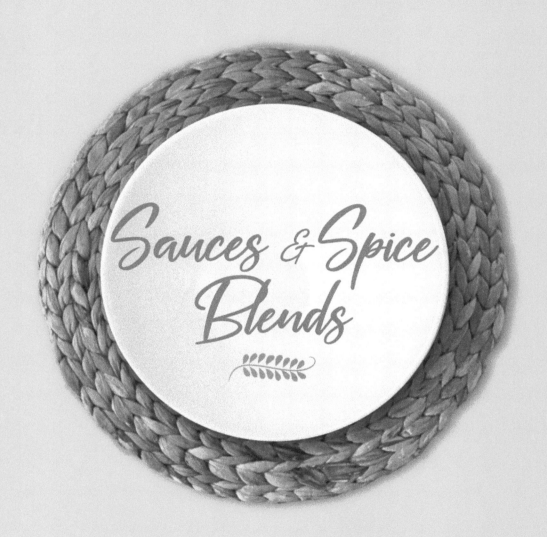

Sauces & Spice Blends

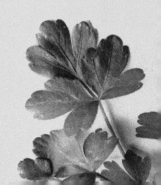

Authentic Niter Kibbeh
(Ethiopian Spiced Clarified Butter)

Makes about 2 cups

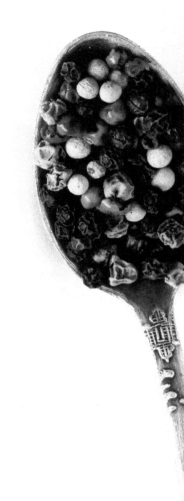

INGREDIENTS:

1 pound unsalted butter, cubed

¼ c chopped yellow onion

3 tbsp minced fresh garlic

2 tbsp minced fresh ginger

1 2-inch cinnamon stick

1 tsp whole black peppercorns

3 BLACK cardamom pods *(not the green cardamom variety)*

3 whole cloves

1 tsp fenugreek seeds

1 tsp coriander seeds

1 tsp dried oregano

½ tsp cumin seeds

¼ tsp ground nutmeg

¼ tsp ground turmeric

1 tbsp besobela (Ethiopian Sacred Basil) *if you can find it, otherwise omit*

1 tbsp kosseret (a sage like plant, wild herb) *if you can find it, otherwise omit*

PREPARATIONS:

1. Toast the whole spices over medium heat in a dry skillet for a few minutes until very fragrant. Be careful not to scorch the spices or they will become bitter. Set aside.

2. Place all the ingredients in a medium saucepan and bring it to an extremely low simmer. Continue to simmer over low for at least one hour or up to 9 minutes. BE VERY CAREFUL NOT TO BURN THE BUTTER. If it burns it will be bitter and there is no salvaging it.

3. Pour everything through a fine-mesh cheesecloth.(No need to skim off the foam, everything will be removed during straining.)

4. Pour the niter kibbeh into a jar, let it cool, and cover so that it is airtight. It will keep at room temperature for several weeks, in the fridge for at least a couple of months, and even longer in the freezer. The aroma is fantastic! It reminds me of my mother's cooking! Probably the quickest way to infuse a number of spices into anything you're going to saute! Truly fantastic, and worth having on hand! It will be harder in the fridge and freezer, so let it come to room temp. for easy scooping)

AWASE

Makes about 1/4 cup

This is a hot condiment that you make with Berbere, it's almost used as an Ethiopian-style ketchup. I f you want to up the heat on you soups and stews, this is what you've been looking for. Can be used to add some heat to any dish, but be careful.

INGREDIENTS:

2 tablespoons Berbere or mild chili powder

1 teaspoon cayenne pepper

1/2 teaspoon ground ginger

1/4 teaspoon ground cardamom, preferably freshly ground

1/2 teaspoon salt

2 tablespoons fresh lemon juice

1 tablespoon dry red wine

1 tablespoon water

1/2 teaspoon olive oil

PREPARATIONS:

1. Combine the first 5 ingredients in a small saute pan. Toast ingredients over medium heat, stirring constantly, until fragrant. About 30 seconds, then remove pan from heat.
2. Whisk in the lemon juice, olive oil, red wine, and water. Let cool afterwards.
3. Store mixture in an airtight container in the refrigerator for 3 to 4 days.

BERBERE

Makes 1 cup

This is a mix of spices that make up the Ethiopian signature taste, known to be used on a variety of dishes.

INGREDIENTS:

1 teaspoon fenugreek seeds

1/2 cup ground dried Serrano chillies or other ground dried chillies

1/2 cup paprika

2 tablespoons salt

2 teaspoons ground ginger

2 teaspoons onion powder

1 teaspoon ground cardamom, preferably freshly ground

1 teaspoon ground nutmeg

1 teaspoon garlic powder

1 teaspoon ground cloves

1/4 teaspoon ground cinnamon

1/4 teaspoon ground allspice

1/4 teaspoon ground coriander

PREPARATIONS:

1. If you can't find fenugreek seeds already ground, finely grind them with a mortar and pestle or in an electric spice/coffee grinder. Stir together with the remaining ingredients in a small bowl until well combined.

2. Store the mixture in an airtight container in the refrigerator, this has a shelf life (refrigerated) for up to 3 months.

Brandon's Steak Marinade

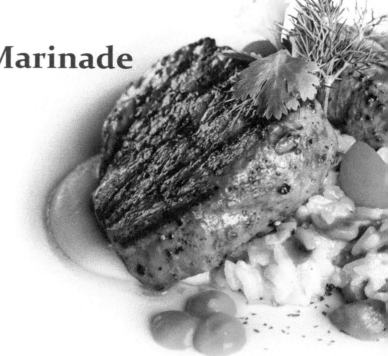

INGREDIENTS:

2 tablespoons honey

2 tablespoons lemon juice

1 teaspoon ground black pepper

1 teaspoon dried rosemary

1 teaspoon minced garlic

1/2 cup soy sauce

1/4 cup olive oil

1/4 cup water

PREPARATIONS:

Pour all ingredients into a pan, place thawed steaks in the pan, cover, and refrigerate for 8 hours. Then cook.

Note: Thawed steaks should marinate in the fridge at least 8 hours, flip over every 4 hours. Frozen steaks should marinate in the fridge for 24 hours, flip around every 12 hours. Grill to preference.

I actually ended up adding 3 ingredients to this family recipe (black pepper, rosemary, and olive oil), just to get the most flavor after the steak was grilled. I'm also a huge fan of rosemary! You can pair this with rosemary potatoes in any way you like potatoes cooked. I've done it with halved baby potatoes drizzled in olive oil and sprinkled with garlic salt and rosemary (350F for 30-45 minutes with one or two shakes of the pan to rotate the potatoes)! You can also do rosemary mashed potatoes and use a sprig of rosemary as decor on top of the finished product. I would suggest something light like asparagus for the greens since meet and potatoes are the main. Good ol' Minnesota meat and potatoes!

CHERMOULA

Makes 1-1/2 cups

Used by cooks particularly in Morocco and Tunisia as a rub for fish, but you can use it with meat or even chicken. It a great blend of citrus and herbs with a small touch of heat.

INGREDIENTS:

8 garlic cloves

1/2 cup smal parsley sprigs

1/3 cup small cilantro sprigs

3/4 teaspoon coriander seeds, ground

Grated zest of 2 lemons

4 teaspoons paprika

2 teaspoons chili powder

2 teaspoons ground cumin

1 cup extra-virgin olive oil

PREPARATIONS:

1. Put the garlic, parsley, cilantro, coriander, lemon zest, paprika, chili powder, and cumin in a blender. Blend on low speed to a coarse puree. While the blender is running, add the oil in a thin & steady stream. Blend until a thick pate forms.

2. Refrigerate in tightly covered container, has shelf life of up to 2 weeks in fridge.

Chimichurri

INGREDIENTS:

1/2 teaspoon fresh lemon juice

1 large bunch cilantro

1 large bunch flat-leaf parsley

1 small shallot, chopped

2 tablespoons oregano

1/2 cup red wine vinegar

1/2 cup apple cider vinegar

2 cups olive oil

6-7 cloves of garlic, minced

Dash of red pepper flakes (if you like a little heat)

Generous servings of salt & pepper to taste

PREPARATIONS:

1. Roughly chop the cilantro, parsley and oregano (including stalks). Place all ingredients in a food processor and pulse, stopping and scraping down sides occasionally until finely minced. Store in refrigerator in a tightly sealed container, has a shelf life of 5 days. Unless freezing, then it's good for a month. A great idea, if you're planning on freezing the Chimichurri sauce, is to use an ice-cube tray. That way you can grab one cube or two if you want to use a little bit of it throughout the month.

Note: Chimichurri sauce is usually served with steak, but you can really use it on any type of protein. You can also put it atop your eggs in the morning for a flavorful breakfast!

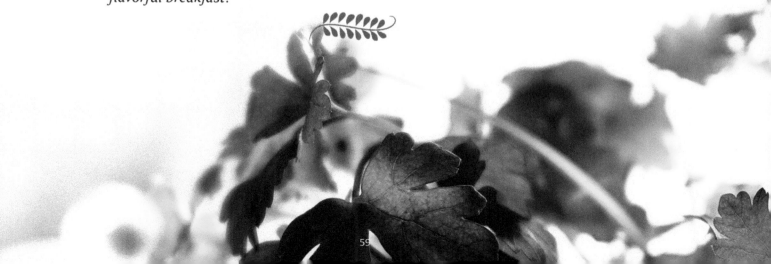

Raspberry Dressing

INGREDIENTS:

2 cups mayo

2/3 cup sugar

1/3 cup Half & Half

1/3 cup raspberry vinegar

Small handful of mint leaves, finely chopped

2 teaspoons Poppyseeds

3 tablespoons raspberry preserves

PREPARATIONS:

1. Mix ingredients together in a bowl.
2. Serve over torn spinach and top with strawberries!

This family recipe is my favorite, especially in the summer! It's great if you want something fresh. I added mint leaves so add more of the freshness factor, and I usually use arugula or a spring mix.

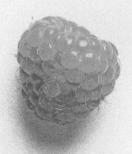

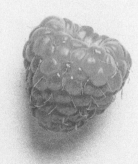

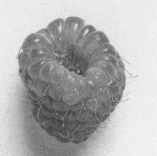

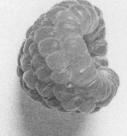

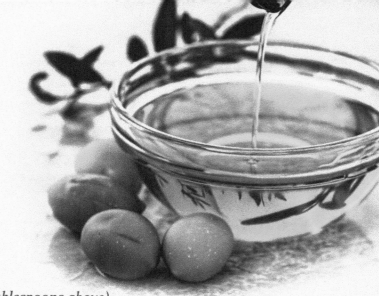

Garem Masala

Makes 1 cup

INGREDIENTS:

1/4 teaspoon mace, ground
(can substitute with nutmeg)

2 tablespoons olive oil

1/2 cup olive oil *(separate from the two tablespoons above)*

One small piece ginger *(fits in palm)* peeled and grated

4 garlic cloves, minced

8 jalapeño chilies, seeds and ribs removed, chopped

1 teaspoon cardamom seeds

 teaspoon ground turmeric

1 teaspoon coriander seeds

2 tablespoons white wine vinegar

PREPARATIONS:

1. In a medium sauce pan, over medium heat, heat 2 tablespoons of the olive oil. Add the ginger, garlic, and jalapeños and sauce until the garlic is golden, about 4 minutes. Add the mace, cardamom, turmeric, and coriander and saute until fragrant, about 1 minute, then remove from the heat.

2. Transfer mixture to blender, add the white wine vinegar, and blend well to combine. Add the remaining 1/2 cup oil in a thin and steady stream while the blender is running on low speed. Blend until well combined.

3. Refrigerated shelf-life is up to 1 week, make sure you store it in an airtight container. Freezer shelf-life is up to 3 weeks.

Rosemary Barbecue Sauce

*Gluten Free

Makes 1-1/4 cups

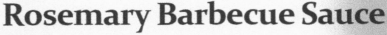

INGREDIENTS:

1 tablespoon olive oil or vegetable oil

1 tablespoon fresh rosemary, finely chopped

1/2 cup finely chopped onion

2 cloves garlic, minced

3/4 cup apple juice

1/2 of. 6-oz can of tomato paste (1/3 cup)

1/4 cup cider vinegar

2 tablespoons packed brown sugar

2 tablespoons molasses

1 tablespoon paprika

1 tablespoon prepared horseradish

1 tablespoon gluten-free Worcestershire sauce, such as Lea & Perrins

1 teaspoon salt

1/2 teaspoon black pepper

PREPARATIONS:

1. In a medium saucepan heat oil over medium, then add onion, garlic and rosemary: cook until onion is tender, stir occasionally. Stir in the remaining ingredients.
2. Bring to mixture to a boil, then reduce heat.
3. Simmer, uncovered, for 30 minutes or until sauce reaches desired consistency. Make sure you're stirring occasionally.

Spicy Peanut Sauce

*Gluten Free

Makes 1-1/4 cups

INGREDIENTS:

1/2 cup cold water

2 teaspoons cornstarch

1/3 creamy peanut butter

1/4 rice vinegar

1/3 cup reduced-sodium Tamari or liquid aminos *(Soy Sauce)*

2 tablespoons honey

1 tablespoon grated fresh ginger

1/4 teaspoon crushed red pepper

1/2 teaspoon lime juice

PREPARATIONS:

1. In a small saucepan whisk cold water and cornstarch, then add in (whisk) the remaining ingredients.
2. Over medium heat, cook and stir until thickened and it bubbles. Continue to cook and stir for 1 minute more.

Uncle Mikey's Teriyaki Marinade

INGREDIENTS:

1 cup lite soy sauce, low sodium

6 – 7 Tbsp brown sugar *(add more if needed, until mixture tastes a bit sweet)*

ADD TO ABOVE, THEN MIX:

2 tsp sesame oil

2 small containers of sesame seeds *(~4 oz)*

½ tsp garlic powder

4 – 6 green onions, chopped *(include green stalks)*

½ tsp black pepper

1 tsp chili powder

PREPARATIONS:

1. Mix together soy sauce and brown sugar.
2. Mix remaining ingredients to soy and brown sugar mix.

This is a great marinade for chicken! You can marinate 6 chicken breasts for about a ½ hour, then grill them! You can use the leftover chicken breasts for UNCLE MIKEY'S CHINESE CHICKEN SALAD, so making more chicken breasts in the marinade would be welcome.

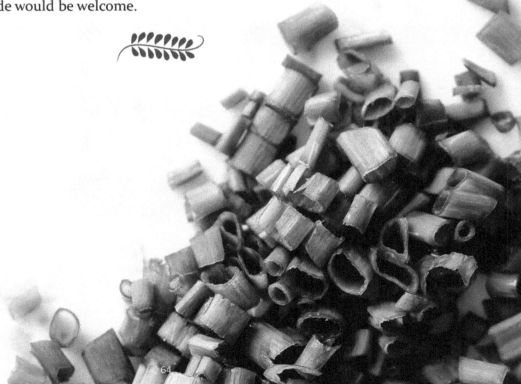

Recipe Notes

Recipe Notes

"

"Carry out a random act of kindness, with no expectation of reward, safe in the knowledge that one day someone might do the same for you. I don't go by the rule book...I lead from the heart, not the head. Family is the most important thing in the world."

- Princess Diana

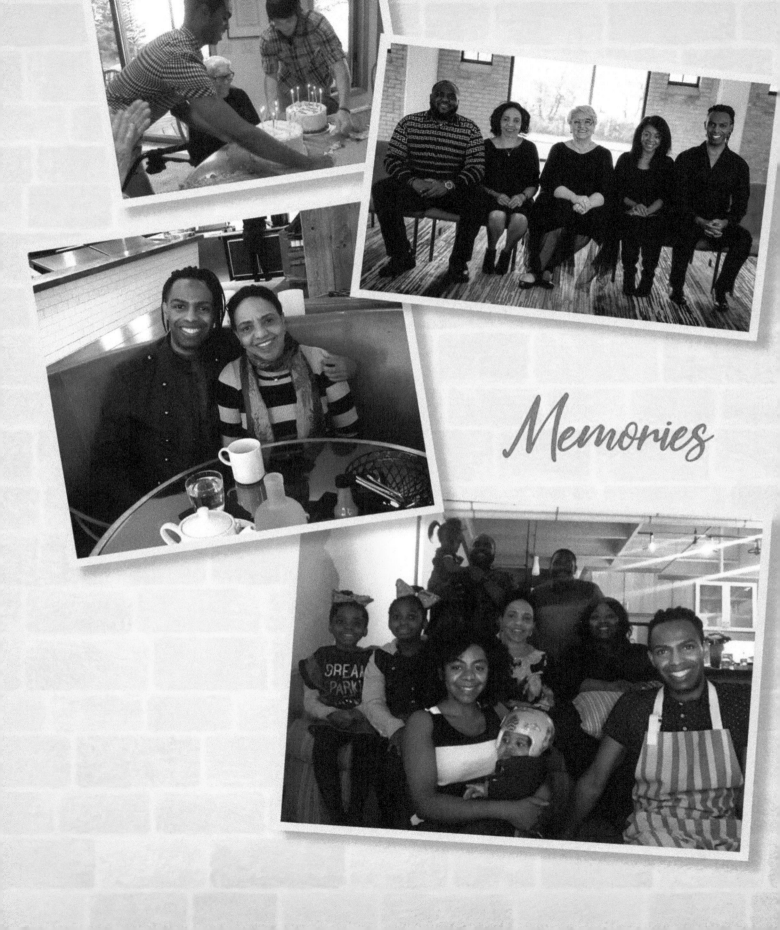

Memories

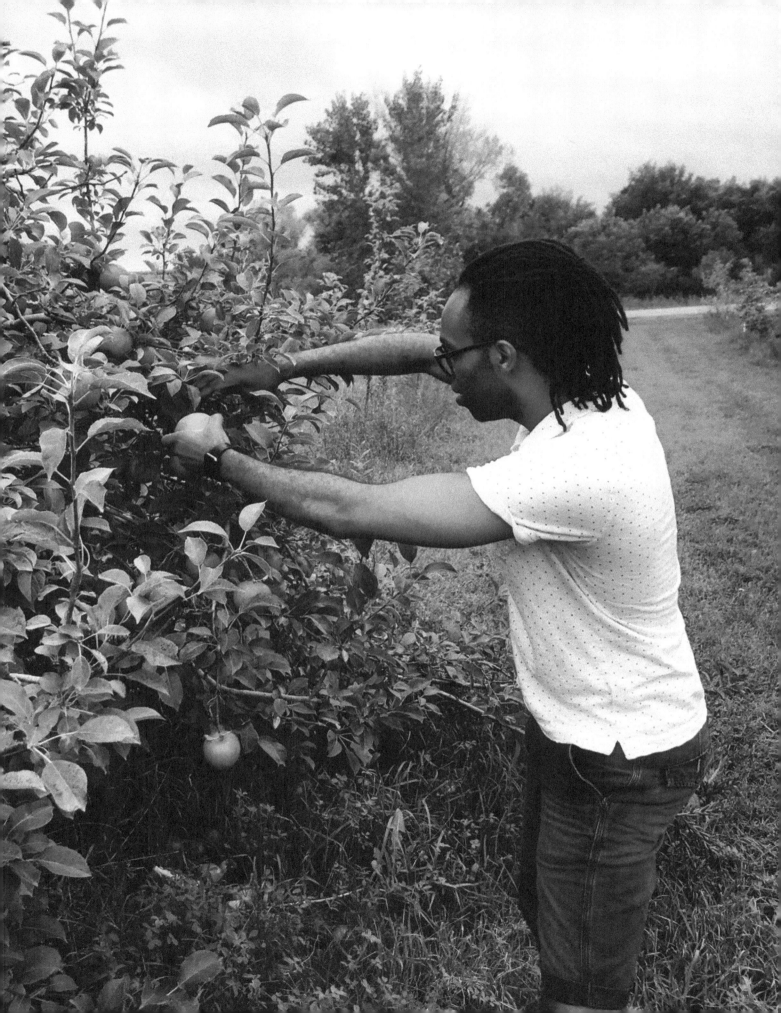

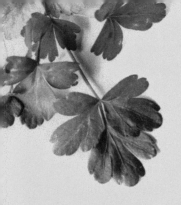
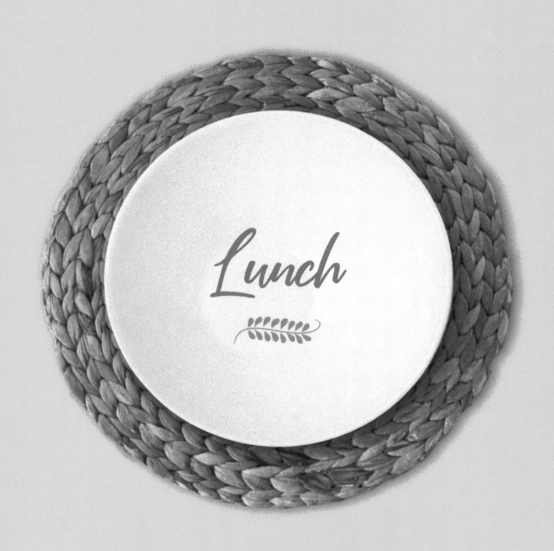

Lunch

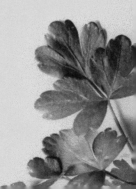

Benny P's BLT's

INGREDIENTS:
1 Large French Bread Loaf
1 Package of Bacon
1/2 cup of mayo
2 tbsp of Tapatio Hot Sauce *(mexican food section at Cub, Lunds, etc)*
Tomatoes
Romaine Lettuce

PREPARATIONS:

1. Cook Bacon the best way you know how, I like over medium high heat on a cast iron skillet.
2. Slice French Loaf into toast-able sections and toast them lightly.
3. Mix the mayo and the Tapatio into a small bowl and spread lightly over the toasted bread.
4. Perfectly cover 1/2 the pieces with Bacon.
5. Perfectly cover the bacon with tomato.
6. Perfectly cover the tomato with lettuce.
7. Place empty pieces of bread over the covered pieces and cut in half.
8. Serve immediately and I dare you to not make a sound when eating them...impossible.

*If you're in the Minnesota area, my cousin Ben recommends the Mexican Style Bacon from Lantto's Store in French Lake, MN. He says "trust me, it's the best you've ever had!"

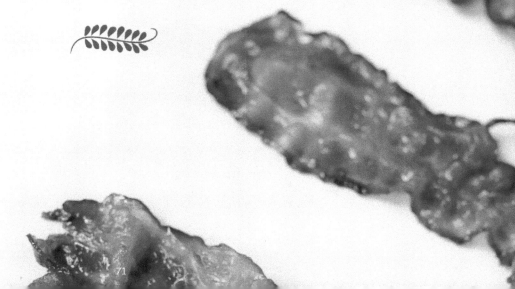

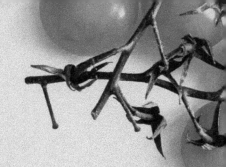

Chix Tinga Tacos *(Chicken)*

Makes 3 servings (about 10-12 tacos)

INGREDIENTS FOR CHICKEN TINGA TACOS:

1 tablespoon olive oil

1 cup roughly chopped sweet onion

2 cloves garlic, minced

1–2 chipotle peppers in adobo sauce, chopped

1 teaspoon dried oregano

1/4 teaspoon rosemary

1/2 teaspoon ground cumin

3/4 cup canned crushed fire-roasted tomatoes

1/4 cup chicken stock

1/2 teaspoon kosher salt

3 cups shredded cooked chicken *(rotisserie chicken works)*

10 (6-inch) corn tortillas

2 ripe avocados, sliced

1/4 cup chopped fresh cilantro

1/2 cup diced red onion

PREPARATIONS:

1. Grab a large skillet and heat it over medium heat. Once hot, pour in the olive oil then pour in the onion. Saute the onion until its tender/softer, then add in the garlic. Should be pretty fragrant. Soon after you should add the oregano and cumin. Let that toast for about 30 seconds.

2. Add tomatoes, the stock, and finally the salt. Cook until it comes to a simmer, roughly 5-6 minutes.

3. Throw chicken into skillet, cover and cook on low heat for about 3-4 minutes with stirring about every minute. You can add salt/pepper/etc for taste at this point.

4. Serve with tortillas, avocado, cilantro, and diced red onion.

* I once made a chipotle sauce to drizzle on top of my taco and it was off the hook! Feel free to replicate this with different proteins, although be careful with fish.

Good ol' Sloppy Joes

Makes 6 servings

INGREDIENTS:

1 pound lean ground beef

1 tablespoon unsalted butter

1/2 yellow onion chopped

1/2 green bell pepper chopped

1 clove garlic minced

2 teaspoons yellow mustard

3/4 cup ketchup

2 tablespoons brown sugar

1/2 teaspoon Kosher salt

1/4 teaspoon ground black pepper

PREPARATIONS:

1. Using a large skillet on medium heat, add oil. Once hot, add in onion, pepper, and garlic. Sauté until onion is tender, then add the ground beef. Stir, then add a little garlic salt. Cover with lid and let it cook for about 30 seconds-1 minute. Stir then let cook without lid 1-2 minutes. Stir then repeat until brown. If there's excess water, there shouldn't be, drain.

2. Add in the rest of the ingredients, stir, then cover for 30 seconds - 1 minute. Uncover, then occasionally stir and cook until the sauce has thickened. At this point you can start adding things for taste.

Serve on buns with any sides you want.

Quick Turkey Burgers

Makes 4 servings

INGREDIENTS:

1 lb. ground turkey

1 large egg, beaten

2 cloves garlic, minced

1 tbsp. Worcestershire sauce
(can substitute soy sauce)

2 tbsp. freshly chopped parsley

Kosher salt

Freshly ground black pepper

1 tbsp. extra-virgin olive oil

Hamburger buns

Arugula

Sliced tomatoes

Mayonnaise *(regular or chipotle)*

PREPARATIONS:

1. First combine turkey, egg, garlic, Worcestershire sauce, and parsley in a large bowl. Season with salt and pepper, then mix.
2. Once mixed, create four flat burger-patties out of the mixture.
3. You'll need a medium sized skillet on medium heat. Heat the olive oil, then add the burger-patties to the skillet. Cook the burger-patties until they're a light golden color, but most importantly cooked through. Should be about 4-5 minutes on each side. Serve on a bun with arugula, sliced tomato, and mayonnaise.

* I'm a huge fan on Rosemary so sometimes I'll do one of two things:

    A. I'll actually throw some Rosemary into the mixture in the bowl.

    B. I'll throw some Rosemary into the oil before placing the patties in there.

I think it gives the turkey a nice flavor.

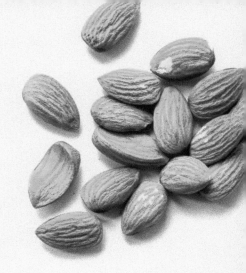

Uncle Mikey's Chinese Chicken Salad

INGREDIENTS:

4 cooked chicken breasts *(from Uncle Mikey's Chicken recipe)*

1 small head cabbage

1 pkg chicken flavored Top Ramen, uncooked

4 – 6 green onions, chopped

2 small containers of sesame seeds (~4 oz)

4 Tbsp slivered almonds, toasted

DRESSING INGREDIENTS:

¼ cup peanut oil

¼ cup sesame oil

6 Tbsp red wine vinegar *(add until mixture is acidic and cuts oil taste)*

1 tsp sugar

½ tsp black pepper

Top Ramen chicken flavor pack

PREPARATIONS:

1. Shred chicken breasts.
2. Cut cabbage into thin strips.
3. Smash Top Ramen noodles. Save flavor pack.
4. Chop green onions (include green stalks).
5. Toss above ingredients with sesame seeds and almonds.

DRESSING PREPARATIONS:

1. Combine remaining ingredients.
2. Keep dressing at room temperature.
3. Toss right before serving.

Recipe Notes

Recipe Notes

"I can do things you cannot, you can do things I cannot; together we ca do great things."

- Mother Teresa

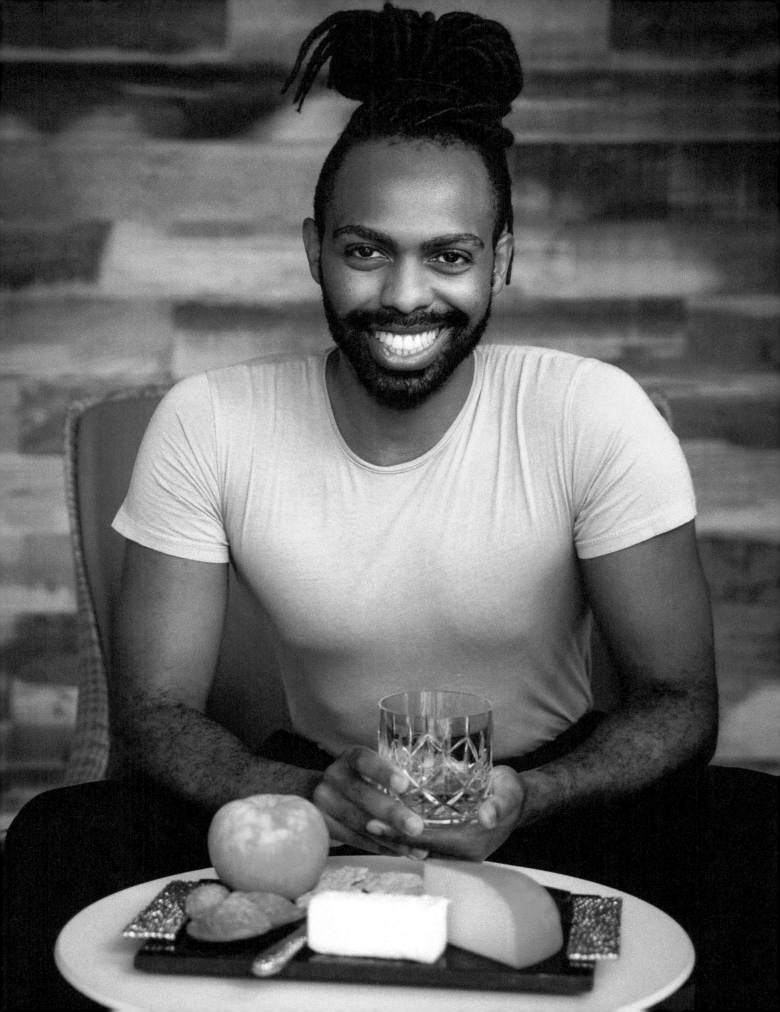

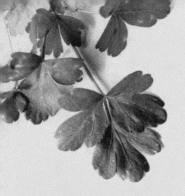
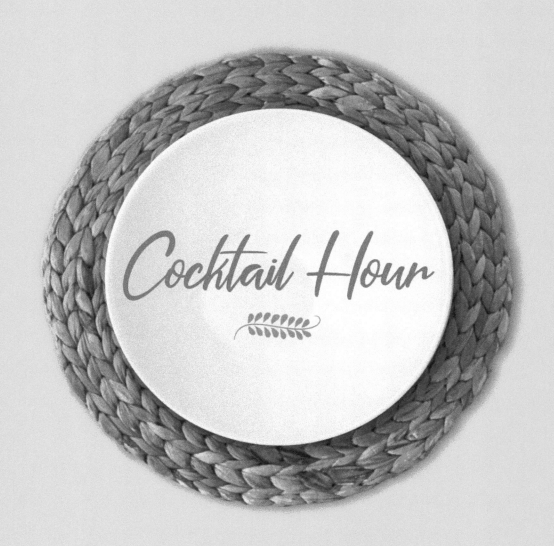

Cocktail Hour

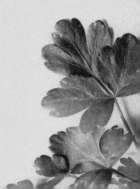

Auntie Ann's Frozen Daiquiris

INGREDIENTS:

1 large frozen lemonade

1 large frozen limeade

1 cup sugar

10 cups water

1 quart Rum

PREPARATIONS:

1. Mix all ingredients together in a bucket (ice cream pale) and put in freezer to freeze.
2. Serve when frozen.

Auntie Ann's Margaritas

INGREDIENTS:

Full bottle of Tequila (Jose Cuervo Silver)

Full bottle of Jose Cuervo margarita mix

Half a bottle of triple sec (Any brand, grand marnier if you're being fancy)

Half a bottle of sweet and sour mix

1 gallon freezer-safe bucket with lid

PREPARATIONS:

1. Mix all ingredients inside bucket, close bucket with lid, and put into freezer.
2. Let freeze overnight or 1-2 days before event.

Green Tea & Peach Julep

Makes 4 servings

INGREDIENTS:

1 cup green tea cooled

1 cup freshly made peach juice

1/4 cup freshly squeezed lemon juice

4 ounces (1/2 cup) good quality bourbon

Fresh mint leaves, lemon slices, and ice cubes *(for garnishing)*

Mixing stick

PREPARATIONS:

1. Have your serving glasses ready with ice in them, pour the amount of bourbon you want in each glass.
2. Mix all the green tea, peach juice, and lemon juice in a pitcher. Mix well with mixing stick.
3. Pour the mix into each glass.
4. Use the lemon slices and fresh mint leaves as garnish. Best when served immediately.

*Sometimes people want this a little sweeter, in which case I would recommend a simple syrup.

Poppy's "Or Something"
Serves 1

INGREDIENTS:

3 shots of Single Malt Scotch *(Any good scotch that he didn't bring)*

Low ball glass

Ice

PREPARATIONS:

1   Add ice to a low ball glass, pour 3 shots of a single malt scotch in it.

Raspuava Mojito *(Raspberry-Guava)*
Serves 1

INGREDIENTS:

5 Fresh Raspberries

1 1/2 tablespoons Simple Syrup

6 pieces Mint Leaves

2 tablespoons Guava Puree

2 1/2 tablespoons of White Rum

Club soda (measurement to taste)

PREPARATIONS:

1.   In a tall glass add raspberries and simple syrup, and muddle.

2.   Add mint leaves, guava puree, and white rum after muddling.

3.   Add ice and cover glass in order to shake, Shake well.

4.   Pour into new glass over ice. Top with club soda.

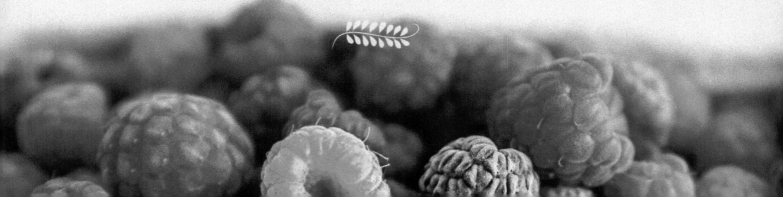

Saba's Bloody Mary

Serves 1

INGREDIENTS:

ZingZang Bloody Mary mix

1 or 2 shots of vodka

2-3 drops of Worcestershire sauce

1 tsp of pickle juice

2-3 drops of Tabasco sauce

Pickles *(optional)*

Olives *(optional)*

A sprinkle of pepper

PREPARATIONS:

1. Fill a tall glass halfway with ice, pour all the above ingredients in glass, stir and serve.

Fresh Arianna's (Watermelon-Mint Mocktail)

Serves 4

INGREDIENTS:

4 cups watermelon, seeded and cubed *(about 3 pounds)*

1/2 cup water

24 mint leaves, divided

8 tablespoons super-fine sugar *(adjust if too sweet when using a naturally sweeter watermelon)*, divided

Ice cubes

PREPARATIONS:

1. Add the watermelon and the water to the blender, and puree until smooth. Divide the mint leaves, sugar, and lime slices among 8 glasses and muddle the ingredients.
2. Add ice to each glass and pour in the watermelon-mint cocktail. Stir and serve.

Mocktail de la Renewed

Serves 4

INGREDIENTS:

9 oz carrot juice

15 oz apple juice

2.25 oz ginger syrup *(1:1 ration ginger juice/sugar)*

.75 oz lime juice

Stir stick

PREPARATIONS:

1. In a large pitcher, add ice then combine all ingredients.
2. Mix well with Stir stick, then pour into glasses.

Recipe Notes

Recipe Notes

"

"Relationships are based on four principles: respect, understanding, acceptance and appreciation."

- Mahatma Gandhi

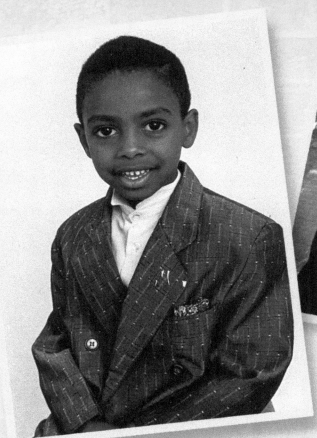

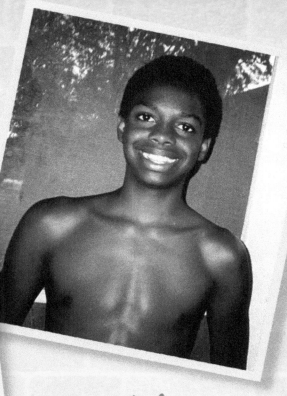

Memories

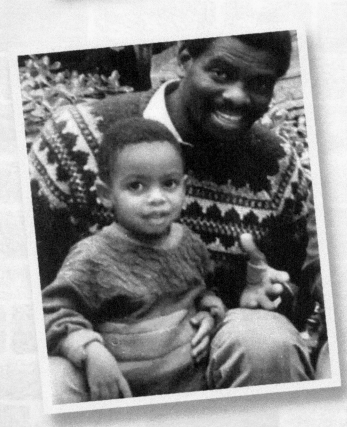

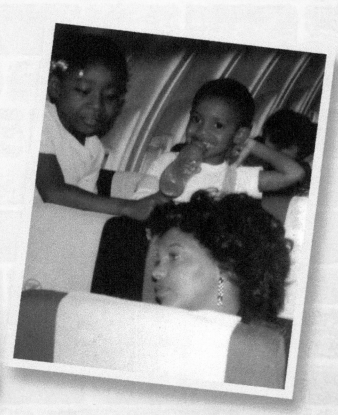

Kasáno

We finally landed in the Minneapolis, Minnesota after our long flights from Lusaka, Zambia.

We made our way down to baggage claim, and got all of our luggage. We were waiting inside for a taxi when I suddenly felt a little hand tug mine a few times. Kasáno looked at me and said "Mom...why do they have refrigerators in the middle of the airport? What if people went inside and it closed? They won't be able to come out!". I was confused, but then realized what he was talking about. I looked at him and through my laughter I answered "Kasáno... that's outside!"

It was so cold outside that he believed everyone exiting the airport was walking into a refrigerator. I can't imagine the stress he was carrying.

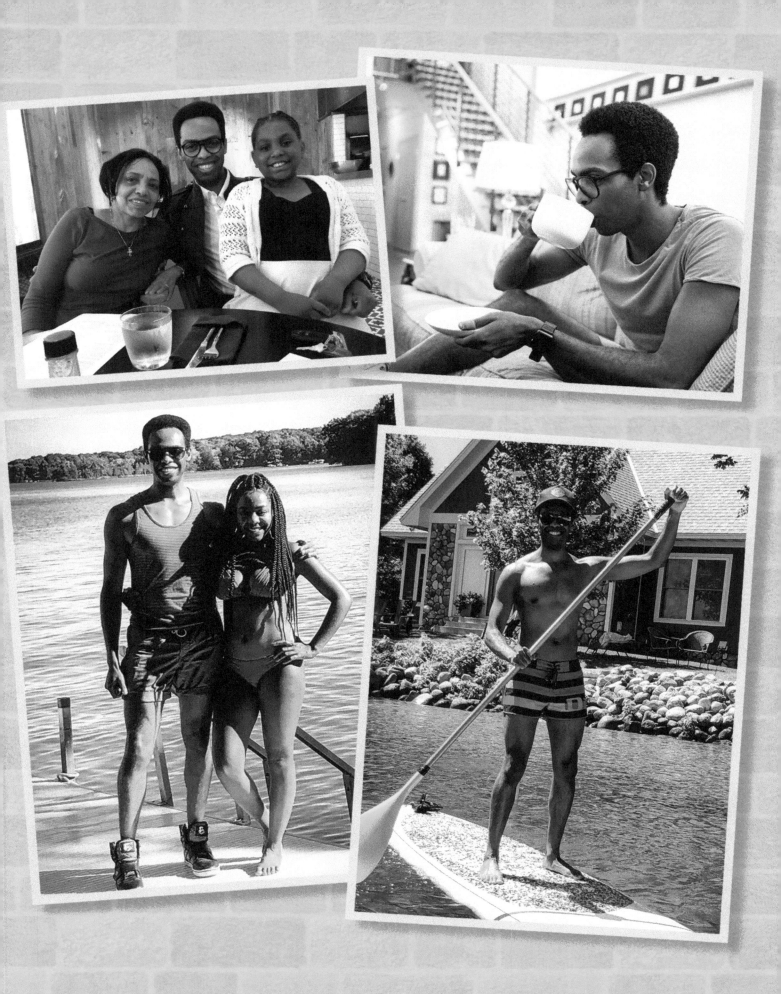

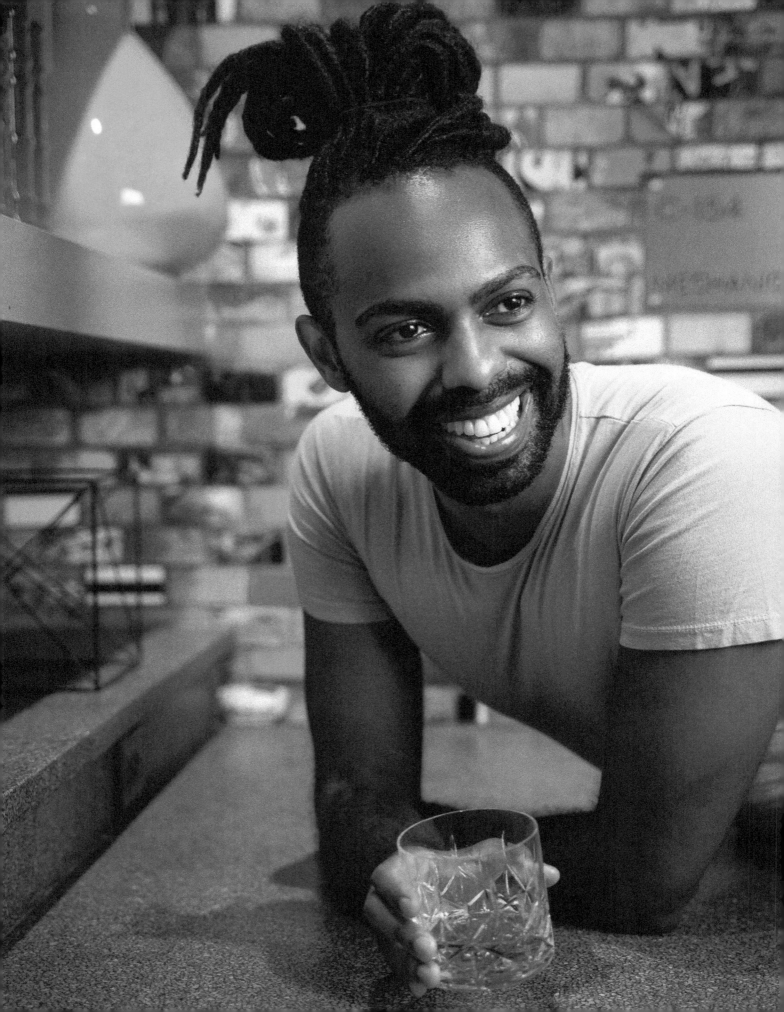

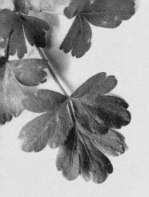
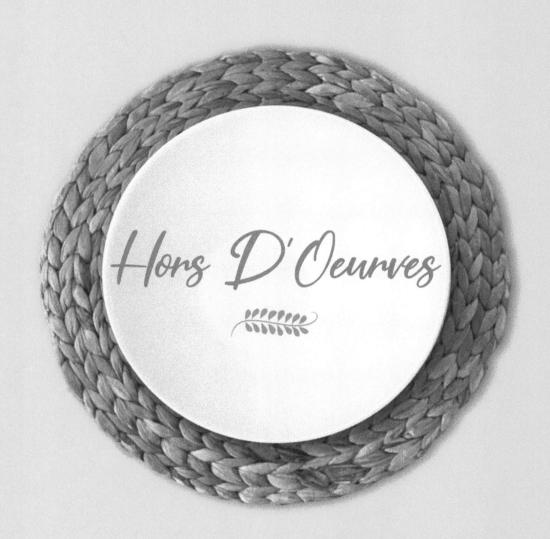

Hors D'Oeurves

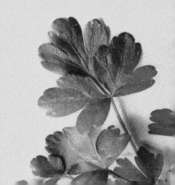

Artichoke Dip

INGREDIENTS:

1 can artichoke hearts, drained and chopped

1/2 cup parmesan cheese *(or more)*

1/2 cup grated cheddar

1/2 cup grated jack cheese

1/2 cup grated mozzarella

1-2 tablespoons parsley

Garlic and onion powder for taste

PREPARATIONS:

1. Mix and bake at 350° for 20 to 25 minutes.

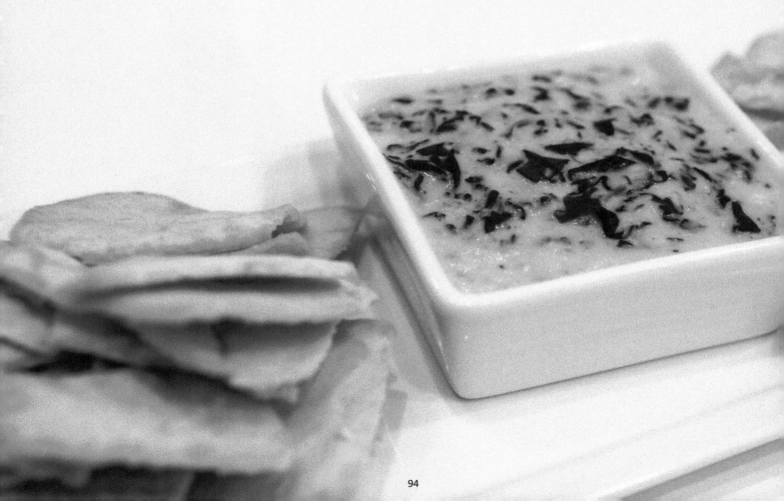

Brie, Fig, and Prosciutto Crostini

Makes 24 Crostini

INGREDIENTS:

1 baguette

1/4 cup extra virgin olive oil

Salt and pepper

8 ounces Brie

4 ounces prosciutto - thinly sliced

1/2 cup fig jam

2 cups baby arugula

1 tablespoon extra virgin olive oil

Salt and pepper

Rosemary

PREPARATIONS:

1. Turn broiler on & get baking sheet ready.
2. Slice your baguette diagonally in order to get that almond shape. Place each piece onto the baking sheet to complete a single layer.
3. Dip a brush in the olive oil and brush each baguette piece with the olive oil, sprinkle the each one with rosemary, pepper, and a little salt.
4. Put the baking sheet in your oven for about 4 minutes, until they look golden. remove from oven and let the cool.
5. Once cool, spread some fig jam on each piece and add prosciutto and brie on top of the jam.
6. In a small bowl, mix the arugula, oil, and a pinch of salt and pepper. Toss to mix. Add a couple pieces of arugula to finish off the presentation.

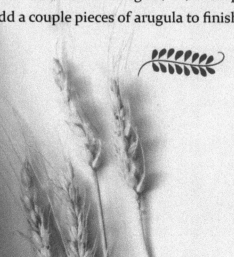

Cowboy Caviar

INGREDIENTS:
1 can garbanzo beans
1 can black beans
1 can corn
2 bell peppers (yellow, orange, or red)
1/2 yellow onion
2 avocado
2 mangos
4 limes juiced
Handful of cilantro
2 teaspoons garlic powder

PREPARATIONS:
1. Drain & rinse garbanzo beans, black beans and corn and toss into large bowl.
2. Cut bell peppers, onion, avocados and mangos into salt cubes and add to the bowl. Stir so ingredients are well mixed.
3. Add lime juice, cilantro and garlic powder and give one more good stir. It will be ready to eat right away, but tastes even better after a few hours in the fridge. Serve with tortilla chips.

*Im a huge fan of the tortilla chips that have a hint of lime, those also go well with this recipe!

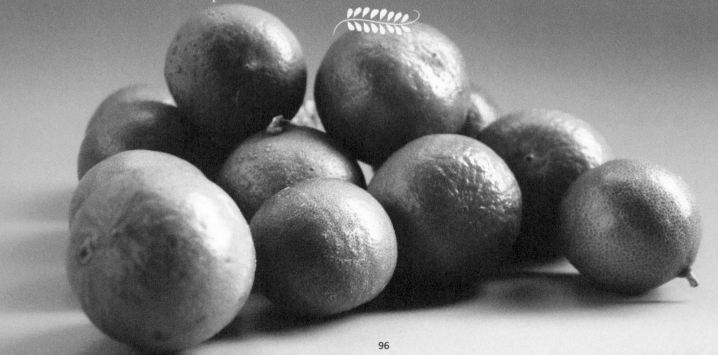

Edena's Dip

INGREDIENTS:

8oz cream cheese

16oz sour cream

Large jar of dried beef, chopped

1/4 green bell pepper

1/4 red bell pepper

1 small onion

PREPARATIONS:

1. Heat in a crockpot or small sauce pot until smooth, creamy, and hot.
2. Serve with your choice of crackers on the side. I recommend Triscuits.

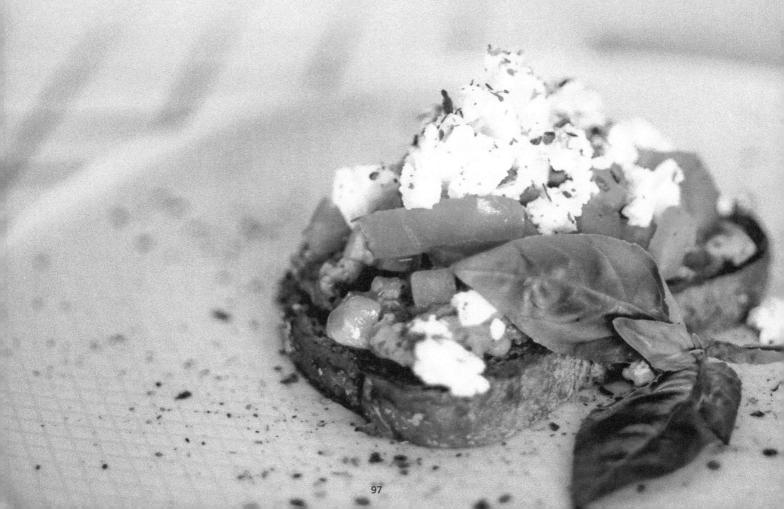

Recipe Notes

Recipe Notes

"

"They say, 'To serve is to love', and I think to serve
is to heal, too."

- Viola Davis

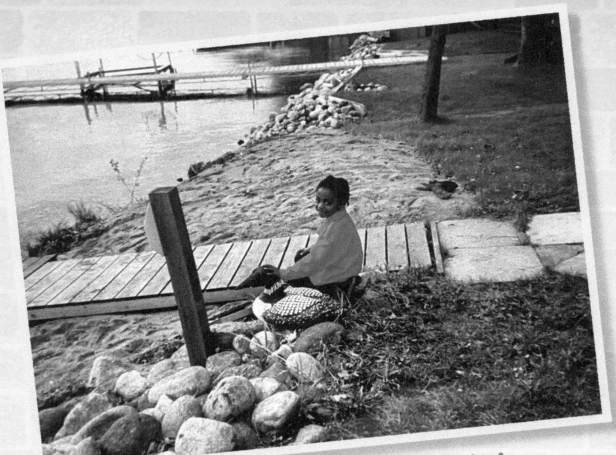

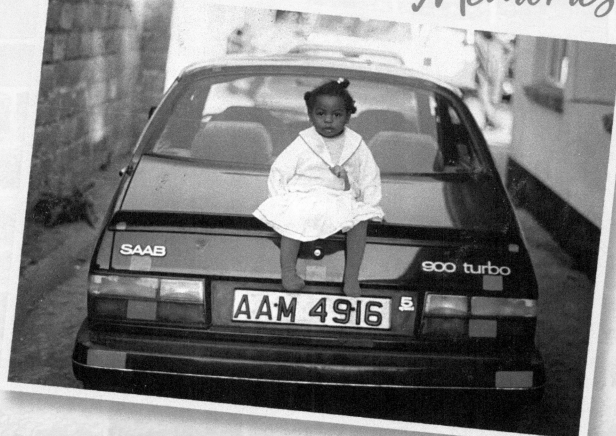

Memories

Dinner Table Stories

Saba

We had no idea if Saba was going to be a girl or a boy, and we were wishing for a girl! As soon as the Saba came out, I immediately was shocked and scared that the she didn't have a face. I was in hysterics, her whole face was black! I remember yelling at the doctor and saying "Oh my God! I drank too much Coca-cola!"

The doctors calmed me down and asked for a pair of scissors. Saba was born with a full head of hair, and so much hair that it covered her whole face. The doctor cut her hair, and it was such a big relief that she had a face!

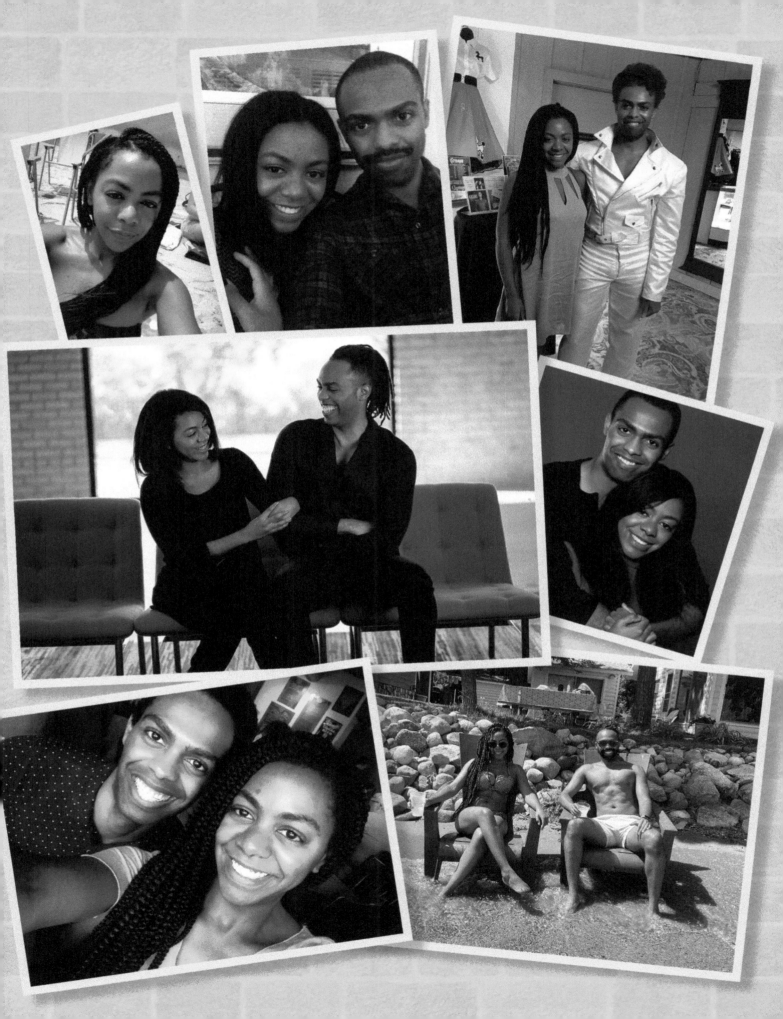

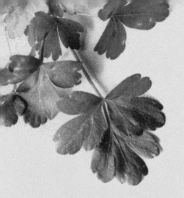
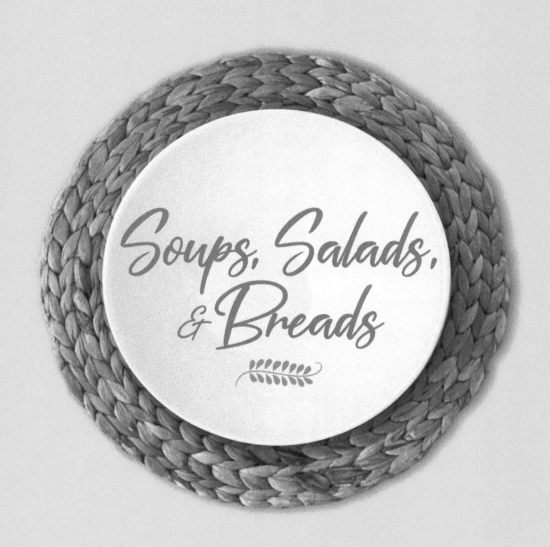

Soups, Salads, & Breads

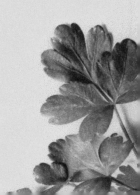

Auntie Ann's Chili Cornbread

Makes 9 servings

INGREDIENTS:

1 cup butter

3/4 cup sugar

4 eggs

1/2 cup diced green chiles

1 1/2 cup creamed corn

1 cup flour

1 cup yellow cornmeal

2 tablespoons baking powder

1 teaspoon salt

1/2 cup shredded cheddar

PREPARATIONS:

1. Preheat the oven to 325°

2. .In a bowl, mix the creamy butter and sugar. Add the eggs one at a time, then add the chilis, corn, and cheese. Mix well together.

3. In a separate bowl combine the dry ingredients, then add the above mixture to it and mix until smooth. Pour into well buttered pan.

4. Bake for about an hour. Enjoy!

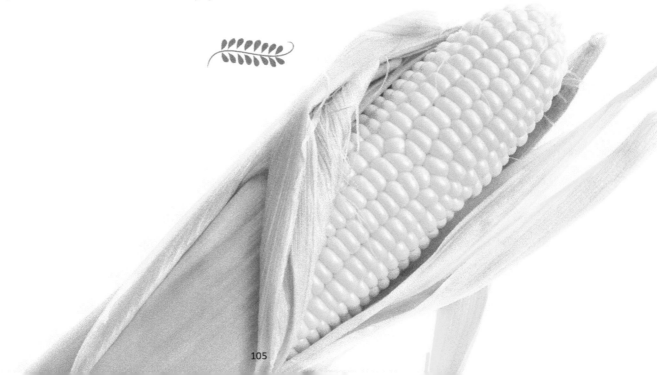

Auntie Ann's Potato Salad

INGREDIENTS:

Eggs, 1 per person

Potatoes, 1 per person

Radishes, 1 for each potato

Salt & pepper for taste

Mayonnaise, enough to help mix

Green onions/scallions

Head of lettuce

PREPARATIONS:

1. Count 1 potato per person, same for eggs, and radishes.
2. In separate pots, boil the eggs and the potatoes. When almost done boiling, break apart head of lettuce and rip into salad pieces. Put it into a big bowl.
3. When eggs and potatoes are ready, peel the potatoes and eggs, and put both in the large bowl.
4. Chop radishes so they're very thin disks, put in bowl.
5. Chop green onion/scallions and put in the bowl.
6. Add mayonnaise to mix it all together. Add salt and pepper for taste. Enjoy.

*I remember eating this salad at the cabin when we would spend entire summers there as kids. Its best when served fresh, and I haven't been able to touch any other potato salad without missing this version. All the kids would help make the salad; one person would chop, the other would peel potatoes, another would peel the egg shells, and one person would tear the lettuce. It certainly can be made by one person, but the memories of cooking it together is what I hold dear to my heart. The outcome made it even more rewarding, to taste something so delicious! Yes I went back for seconds, and most times it was the biggest portion on my plate!

Injera
Makes 12 flatbreads

Make sure to have already made clarified
butter before starting (*look below for butter instructions*)

INGREDIENTS:

1 cup all-purpose flour

2 cups teff flour or whole-wheat flour (*don't use stone-ground flour*)

1 1/2 teaspoons baking powder

1 teaspoon salt

1/2 cup plain yogurt

3 cups club soda

2 tablespoons clarified butter (*see below*)

PREPARATIONS FOR CLARIFIED BUTTER:

1. In a Saucepan, take about 1/2 pound of butter and heat at medium heat.
   Don't stir, wait for the milk fats to separate. It should fall to the bottom.
2. Remove the foam from the top, carefully.
3. Pour the liquid butter, which should be golden, in a container whilst leaving
   the milk solids in the pan. What's in the container should be good for about
   a month when refrigerated.

PREPARATIONS FOR INJERA:

1. Have a large bowl and a smaller bowl ready.
2. In the large bowl, whisk together the teff, flour, baking soda, and salt.
3. In the separate smaller bowl, whisk the yogurt in the club soda. Once mixed,
   stir it into the flour mixture to make a thin, but also smooth batter. If there
   are any lumps, make sure you strain it through a sieve or strainer.
4. Grease a large skillet with clarified butter and heat over medium-high heat.
5. Pour 1/2 cup of batter into the pan in a spiral, starting at the center, and cook
   for an additional 30 seconds. Transfer to a plate and cover with a cloth to keep
   the Injera warm while you cook the remaining batter.

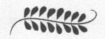

Kale & Sausage Soup

Makes 4-5 servings

INGREDIENTS:

1-2 onions

8-12 cloves garlic

Garlic powder

2 cups Mushrooms, chopped

1 qt chicken stock (more if preferred)

2 lbs Ground sweet Italian sausage, pork or mix of turkey & pork

1 tablespoon ground fennel

2 cups Kale, chopped

Parmesan or soft goat cheese

1 1/2 tablespoonsOlive oil

Salt (For taste)

1 tablespoon Paprika

PREPARATIONS:

1. In a pot, boil your ground sausage until cooked all the way through. Strain and set aside.

2. In a soup pot add olive oil, when oil is hot add onions and cloves of garlic (be generous with the garlic). After a minute or two, stir in chopped mushrooms. Shortly after, add some garlic salt, paprika, and ground fennel. Stir. At this point the onion should be tender and the mixture should be fragrant.

3. Add a quart or more of chicken stock. Bring to a simmer for 10-20 minutes.

4. Taste the broth, feel free to add garlic salt for taste.

5. Towards the end of your 10-20 minute simmer, add the chopped kale an turn off the heat. The temperature of the soup should be hot enough to just blanch the kale.

6. Serve with fresh Parmesan cheese or soft goat cheese.

* For the sausage I would get a ground sweet Italian sausage. You can use a pork or mix of turkey and pork. If you can't find a ground sweet Italian sausage, you can make your own by mixing the sausage with salt, garlic, ground fennel seed, chili flake for spice, black pepper, and paprika. To get more flavor and punch out of it, let it marinate overnight. You can add a teaspoon of fresh squeezed lemon juice to each soup bowl once it's been served if you're looking for a bit of a zing. Sometimes, when boiling the pork, there is a layer of fat from the pork sausage and you'll want to scoop that off with a spoon since it will prevent you from tasting the broth. DISCLAIMER: You will smell like garlic, but its so tasty you'll come back for another bowl! A huge thank you to Aleks K. for this recipe, with a couple changes it has become one of my favorites!

Mindy's Taco Salad

INGREDIENTS:

1 1/2 lbs ground beef browned and rinsed
in cold water

1 15oz. can tomato sauce

1 small onion, chopped

1 tablespoon olive oil

1 pkg. taco seasoning

1 head or bag of shredded lettuce

1 small can sliced olives

1 15oz. can red kidney beans, rinsed and drained

1 tomato

2 cups grated cheese

1 small bottle of Catalina salad dressing

1 bag of regular Fritos

PREPARATIONS:

1. Heat a medium size pan, add olive oil when pan is hot, then throw in the onions. Saute until the onion starts to get tender.

2. Add the ground beef, cook until brown. I usually throw in a couple pinches of garlic salt when doing this, but that's optional.

3. Once browned add the tomato sauce and the taco seasoning, drop the heat a little so it can simmer for about 15 minutes. I sometimes turn up the heat towards the end just to make the sauce thicker a little quicker. Let cool afterwards.

4. In a separate bowl add your lettuce, olives, beans, and add some of the meat from the pan.

5. If you're serving this right away, add the cheese, Catalina dressing and Fritos right away.

*Lately I've been using a spring mix or arugula instead of shredded lettuce, instead of cheese I use avocado, and instead of Fritos I'll use pieces of "a hint of lime" Tostito chips just for a quick lime flavor.

Steak & Bleu Cheese Salad

Makes 4 servings

INGREDIENTS:

12oz lean steak

1 tablespoon olive oil

4 shallots, sliced

1 tablespoon yellow curry powder

INGREDIENTS FOR DRESSING:

1 tablespoon lemon juice

1/2 teaspoon Dijon mustard

1/2 teaspoon Worcestershire sauce

Pinch of salt

INGREDIENTS FOR SALAD:

6 cups mixed greens

2 oz bleu cheese

PREPARATIONS:

1. Rub your steak with garlic salt, pepper, and just a pinch of yellow curry powder on both sides.
2. Heat a medium sized skillet on medium high heat, once hot add the olive oil. Add the steaks and cook each one for about five minute each or until medium-rare (longer if you like your meat done well-cooked). Remove when done and place on chopping board.
3. With heat still on, add shallots or onions to the skillet. I usually add a pinch of garlic salt, pinch of pepper, and a pinch of yellow curry as I saute the shallots/onions. Saute until tender, turn heat off, but leave the shallots/onions in the skillet.
4. In a separate small bowl, add all your dressing ingredients and whisk them together. Set aside when done.
5. Thinly slice the steak, thin enough so you can rip it in half with a bite. Set aside.
6. On a plate or medium bowl, put your mixed greens in first, then the sliced steak, then your shallots/onions, add dressing (you can drizzle, I usually use a tablespoon to drizzle), then sprinkle your bleu cheese last. Enjoy!

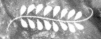

Uncle Mike's Eggs and Noodles

Makes 2 servings

INGREDIENTS:

1 package Chicken Top Ramen noodles with flavor packet

2 cups of water

4 eggs, slightly beaten

½ cup frozen peas (optional)

½ cup chopped ham or chicken (optional)

PREPARATIONS:

1. Add water and peas to a pot and bring to a boil.
2. Breakup the Top Ramen noodles into quarters and add to the water, saving the flavor packet.
3. Continue breaking the noodles up as they soften for approximately 2 min.
4. Add the 4 slightly beaten eggs, stirring the mixture until it comes to a soft boil.
5. Turn off heat and mix in the flavor packet.

Serve this with buttered bread for dipping, you won't regret it!

This is my uncle Mike's recipe. It's so simple and it brings a smile to my face every time. I'm sure there's a way to upgrade this recipe with all sorts of additions and chicken stock, but sometimes it's best to stick to the original. The taste will always bring back memories.

Zambian Chapati

Makes 4 servings

INGREDIENTS:

2 cups all-purpose flour

Salt to taste

Warm water to knead

2 medium onions, chopped/diced

3/4 teaspoon baking soda

Cooking oil *(Peanut oil)*

Mortar & Pestle

Brush *(for oil)*

PREPARATIONS:

1. Wash hands!
2. In a large/wide bowl, sift the flour, baking soda, and salt together then set aside.
3. You'll want to pound the onion in a mortar until the onion is partly a paste, then add this to the bowl of sifted ingredients. Mix together.
4. Slowly add water and knead the dough until the dough becomes soft/well kneaded.
5. Cover the dough with a cloth and let it rest for about half an hour.
6. Divide the the dough into tennis balls sized portions.
7. You'll want to dust each one well with flour once you have them portioned.
8. Using a rolling pin, roll each ball out into discs shapes.
9. Heat a large frying pan, add peanut oil and bring the oil to a simmer. Once the oil is hot, add the discs and cook for a couple of minutes. When you see bubbles coming up, flip the disc over and wait to see the bubbles again. With a brush, apply cooking oil on both sides of the disk and cook until both sides have a golden brown to them. Done!

* You would serve this with a side dish that just came off the stove.

Recipe Notes

Recipe Notes

"Real value isn't in what you own, drive, wear or live. The greater value is found in love and life, health and strength, friends and family!"

- T. D. Jakes

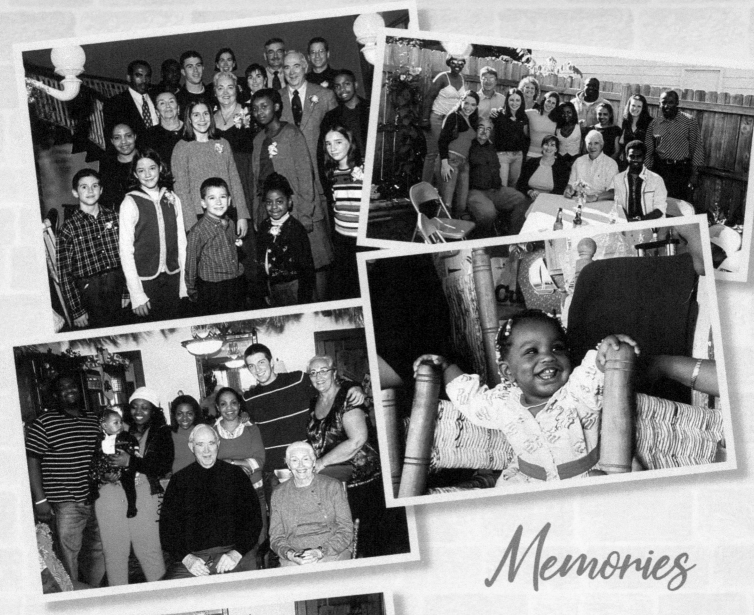

Memories

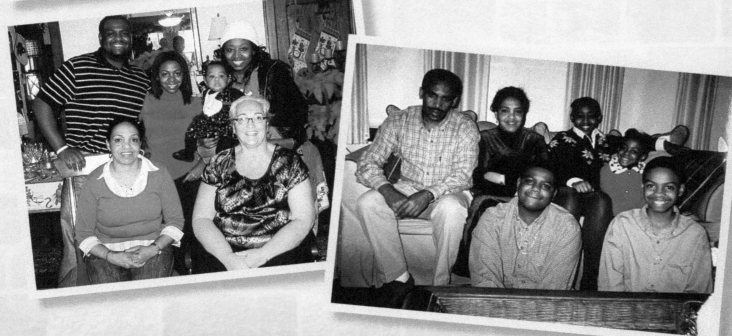

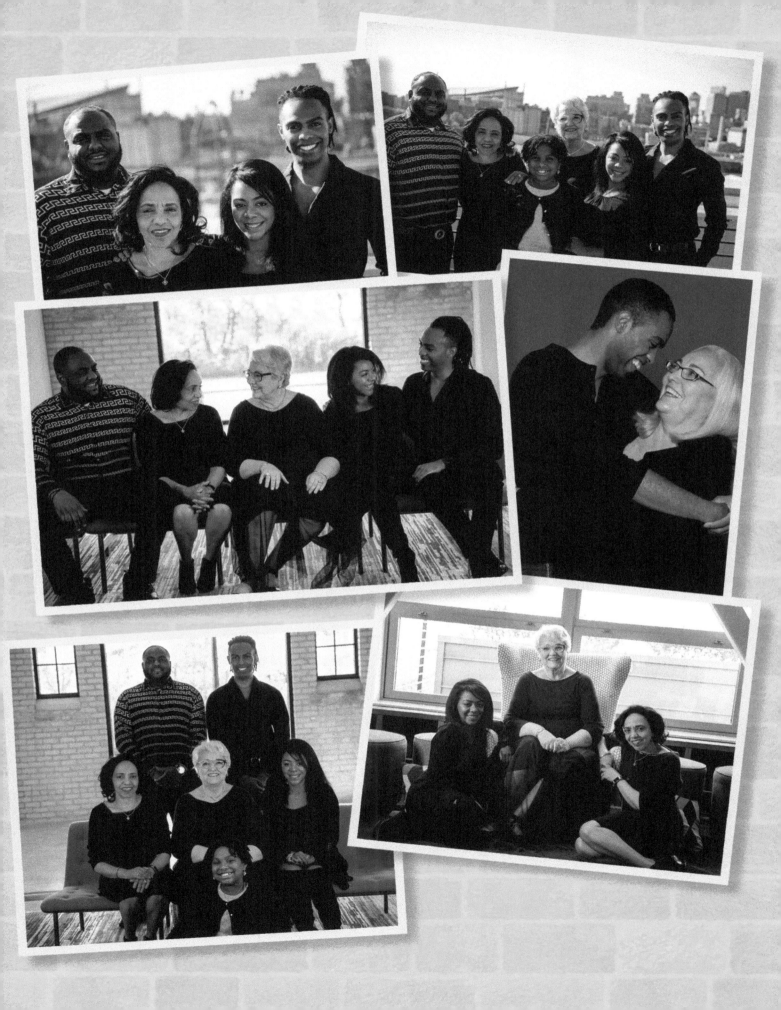

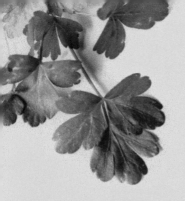
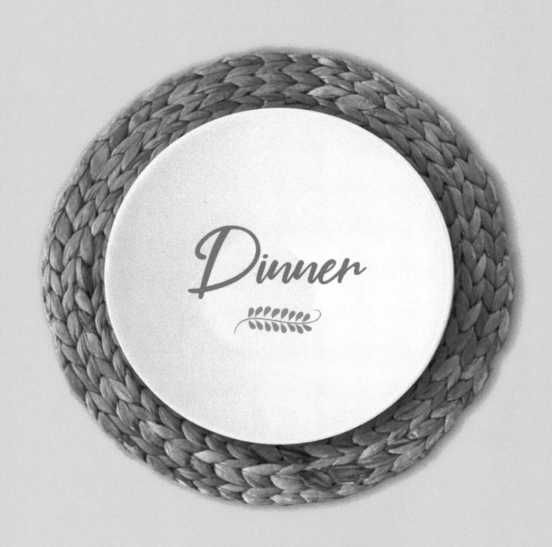
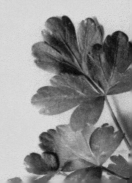

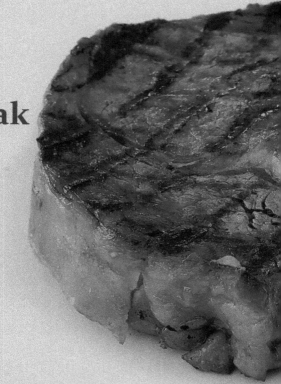

7152 WAGYU Ribeyes Steak

(Medium-rare)

INGREDIENTS:

1.5 in. thick Lunds Wagyu ribeyes *(as many as needed)*

3 tbsp of salted butter

2 tbsp of soy sauce

Salt

Pepper

Olive oil

PREPARATIONS:

1. Preheat oven to 350°.
2. On a baking sheet, place Ribeyes evenly spaced. Salt and pepper liberally on both sides and lightly drizzle olive oil over all of them.
3. Place in oven and bake for 12 minutes.
4. Around the 10 minutes mark, place 1/2 of the butter in the bottom of a frying pan (cast iron preferred) and melt butter until it covers the bottom of the pan.
5. Remove steaks at 12 minutes and quickly place in the hot pan. Cook one side for 30 seconds. When you flip to side two of the steak place the other half of the butter and soy sauce into the bottom of the pan. Baste the steaks with the soy butter sauce for the remaining 30 seconds.
6. Remove from the pan and rest for 1-2 minutes. Enjoy!

*This simple but great recipe is my cousin Ben's recipe, and if you're a fan of a good steak this will have you salivating as you cook it! Sometimes I skip the butter and just use olive oil, and sometimes I skip the soy sauce and use garlic salt. Im in the midst of trying infused olive oils with basil or rosemary, just to give it a subtle pop in flavor. Enjoy!

Charlie's Baked Fish

INGREDIENTS:

Fillets of fish

Butter

Garlic powder

Dill weed

Ground pepper

Mayonnaise

Parmesan Cheese

Lemon Slices

Paprika

PREPARATIONS:

1. Preheat the oven to 400°
2. Arrange the fillets on flat pan and add 3 pats/slices of butter between each fillet.
3. Sprinkle garlic powder, dill weed, and pepper on each fillet.
4. Put about a teaspoon of mayonnaise on each fillet
5. Sprinkle parmesan cheese all over, and add a lemon slice to each fillet and some paprika.
6. Bake at 400° for 15 minutes

*I'm a huge fan of this recipe, sometimes I switch it up.

Here are a few different ways I make it:

1. Ditch the dill and use rosemary and basil.
2. Skip the mayonnaise and use a brush to lightly brush extra virgin olive oil on each fillet.
3. Ditch the dill and use yellow curry powder, skip the lemon slice in this case.

Doro Wett Ethiopian Chicken Stew

Makes 6 servings

INGREDIENTS:

2 small red onions, diced
Salt
1/4 cup Spiced Butter *(look at Ethiopian butter in "Sauces & Spice Blends")*
1/4 teaspoon freshly ground black pepper
Italian Sauce *(Tomato, Basil, Garlic)*, **a whole bottle**
2 garlic cloves, finely chopped *(Optional)*
One 1 1/2-inch piece ginger, peeled and chopped *(Optional)*
1 tablespoon Berbere *(look in "Sauces & Spice Blends")*
2 1/2 cups chicken stock, divided
One 4-to-5-pound chicken, cut into 10 pieces *(don't use wings)*
2 hard boiled eggs, peeled
*Usually it depends on how many people are eating, you would do 1 boiled egg and 1 piece of chicken per person.

PREPARATIONS:

1. In a large deep pot over low heat, combine the onions, a pinch of salt, and pinch of black pepper. Stirring occasionally, cook until the onions loosen (should be about 5 minutes). Add a little water if it starts to stick to the bottom.

2. Add the ginger and garlic and stir until the onions tender. Add a little water if it begins to stick on the bottom.

3. Add the whole bottle of tomato sauce and Berbere. Stir, then wait for it to become thick (let it boil). Then add the Ethiopian butter and mix it well by stirring. Occasionally stir so the sauce gets thick, add a little water if it's sticking to the pot.

4. Add all the chicken to the deep pot. Bring to a simmer for 15 minutes with the occasional stir. Again if it's sticking to the sides or the bottom, add a little water. Adding water will always elongate your simmer time. Once the chicken has cooked, check for taste. Add salt or pepper for taste.

5. Slice the side of each boiled egg on four sides without cutting through.

6. Gently stir in the eggs, the idea is to get the eggs to the bottom of the pot without breaking them. Cover with lid and simmer for another 2 minutes. Turn the heat off and enjoy!

* FYI: This is a fragrant dish and its very delicious! I remember going to school as a kid and anytime a gust of wind would hit me I could smell the Doro Wett! This is the family favorite!

Edena's Peanut Butter Kebabs

INGREDIENTS:

Beef or chicken, chopped into skewer chunks

Green or red bell peppers, chopped into skewer chunks

Sweet or Yellow onion, quartered skewer chunks

Peanut butter (creamy)

Ground back pepper

Garlic Powder

Paprika

Salt

Olive oil

Wooden skewer sticks

Water

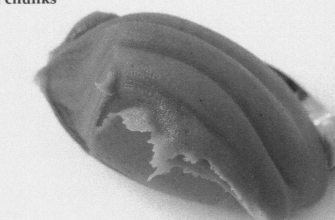

PREPARATIONS:

1. Place all wooden skewers in a pan and soak in olive oil, leave there until you're ready to put meat on the skewer.
2. In a large bowl, mix the beef or chicken with ground pepper, garlic powder, paprika, and salt. Put aside.
3. Quarter the onions (cut into 4) and operate so you have triangle pieces of onion. Put aside.
4. In a small pot, add peanut butter and a little water. Whisk on low heat until it has a bit of a sauce consistency. Pour whisked peanut butter mixture into bowl with meat, and mix.
5. Align the skewer in the following order: Onion, meat, pepper, meat.
6. Grill and enjoy!

Ethiopian Cabbage, Carrots, and Potatoes

INGREDIENTS:

½ **cup olive oil** *(can use less for healthier option)*

4 carrots, thinly sliced

1 onion, thinly sliced

1 tsp sea salt *(may add more at end to your liking)*

½ **tsp ground black pepper** *(I never measure this, I know I use more than ½ tsp!)*

½ - 1 **tsp ground cumin**

¼ - ½ **tsp ground turmeric**

½ **head cabbage, shredded**

5 white potatoes, peeled, cut into 1-inch cubes

PREPARATIONS:

1. Heat olive oil in skillet over medium heat.
2. Cook carrots and onion in oil for about 5 minutes. Stir in the salt, pepper, cumin, turmeric and cabbage and cook 15-20 minutes.
3. Add the potatoes, cover. Reduce heat to medium-low and cook until potatoes are soft, 20-30 minutes.
4. Serve with injera bread Enjoy!

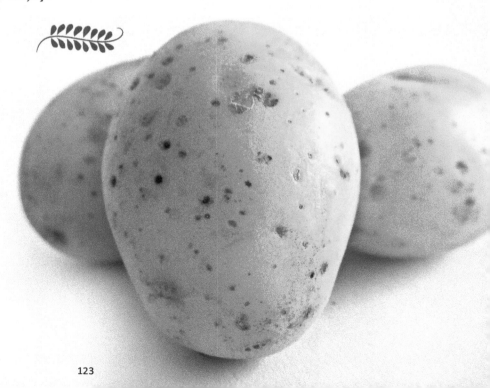

Fool Proof Bride's Dinner

Makes 4 servings

INGREDIENTS:

5 slices of day-old bread

1 egg yolk, beaten

1 tablespoon melted butter

1/2 teaspoon salt

1/8 teaspoon pepper

1/2 teaspoon poultry seasoning

1 teaspoon grated onion

4 pork chops, 1 inch thick

4 meal baking apples, Harrison Apples

1/4 cup seedless raisins

4 tablespoons sugar

1/4 teaspoon cinnamon

4 medium sweet potatoes

3 tablespoons melted butter

PREPARATIONS:

1. Combine bread crumbs, egg yolks, butter, seasonings, and onion to create stuffing. Shape into 4 balls and put aside.
2. Roll sweet potatoes in melted butter, place in shallow pan. Sprinkle with salt and pepper.
3. Place chops in the same baking pan, sprinkle with salt and pepper. Place one ball of stuffing on each chop.
4. Core the apples 3/4 through making sure the center and seeds are out. Also the the bottom is still somewhat intact. Set apples in pan with chops. In a separate bowl combine raisins, sugar, and cinnamon. Fill centers of apples with this mixture.
5. Bake in oven for 1 1/2 hours at about 350°.

Melanzano *(Eggplant)* and Mozzarella Pasta

Makes 4 servings

INGREDIENTS:

1/4 - 1/3 cup extra virgin olive oil

4 cups eggplant (1 large firm eggplant) - *Cut skin off and chop into 1-inch cubes*

16 kalamata olives – pitted and diced

1 large bottle pasta sauce - Classico Mushroom & Ripe Olives *(or your favorite)*

1 - 14 oz can stewed tomatoes, Italian style

3 or 4 sweet Italian sausages (optional) – cooked, remove skin and crumble

8 oz mozzarella cheese – chop into 1 inch cubes

Penne pasta, 16 oz

PREPARATIONS:

1. Put olive oil in large skillet and heat on medium, add eggplant to skillet and cook for about 4 – 5 minutes

2. Add pasta sauce and stewed tomatoes to skillet, and add crumbled sweet Italian sausage. Turn heat to low and simmer.

3. Cook pasta, drain well and add back to pot.

4. Pour simmering sauce into pasta pot.

5. Fold in the kalamata olives and mozzarella cheese cubes until the cheese starts getting stringy. Enjoy!

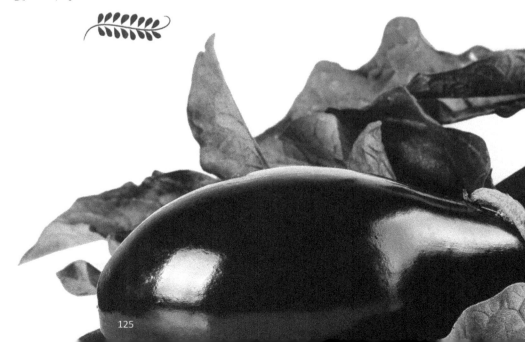

Moroccan Vegetable Tagine

INGREDIENTS:

¼ cup Extra Virgin Olive Oil *(can omit for a healthier version)*

2 medium yellow onions, chopped

8 garlic cloves

2 large carrots, chopped

2 large white potatoes, cubed

1 large sweet potato, cubed

1 tablespoon harissa spice blend

1 teaspoon coriander

1 teaspoon ground cinnamon *(or 1 stick of cinnamon)*

½ teaspoon ground turmeric

2 cup canned tomatoes *(fresh works as well)*

½ cup chopped dried apricot *(prunes or raisins optional)*

1-quart vegetable broth

2 cups cooked chickpeas

1 lemon *(juice of)*

1 handful of fresh parsley leaves

Salt, black pepper

PREPARATIONS:

1. In a large heavy pot or Dutch Oven, heat olive oil over medium heat. Add onions and sauté for 5 minutes, stirring frequently.
2. Add garlic and all chopped veggies
3. Season with salt, black pepper and spices. Toss and stir to combine.
4. Cook for 5-7 minutes on medium-high heat, mixing regularly
5. Add tomatoes, apricots (prunes, raisins).
6. Keep heat on medium-high, cook for 10 minutes.
7. Then reduce heat, cover and simmer for 20-25 minutes or until veggies are tender.
8. Stir in chickpeas, cook another 5 minutes on low heat.
9. Stir in lemon juice and fresh parsley. Taste and adjust seasoning, adding more salt and pepper to your liking.
10. Serve over cous cous or with a nice crusty French bread.

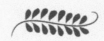

Roasted Chicken Thighs & Peppers

INGREDIENTS:

8 chicken thighs *(about 2 1/2 pounds)*

4 to 6 cloves of garlic, halved

3 new potatoes, quartered

1 red bell pepper, seeded and cut lengthwise into 1/2 -inch strips

1 green bell-pepper, seeded and cut lengthwise into 1/2 -inch strips

1 yellow onion, quartered and cut into 1-inch wedges

1 tablespoon olive oil

1/2 teaspoon dried thyme

1/2 teaspoon salt

Freshly ground pepper to taste

PREPARATIONS:

1. Preheat oven to 425°.
2. Toss all ingredients in a 9-by-13-inch baking dish lightly coated with cooking spray or oil. Spread out ingredients in a single layer.
3. Roast uncovered until vegetables are tender-crisp, about 30 minutes. Turn chicken and vegetables and cook until chicken is no longer pink in the center, 15 to 20 minutes longer. Arrange on a heated platter and serve immediately. Enjoy!

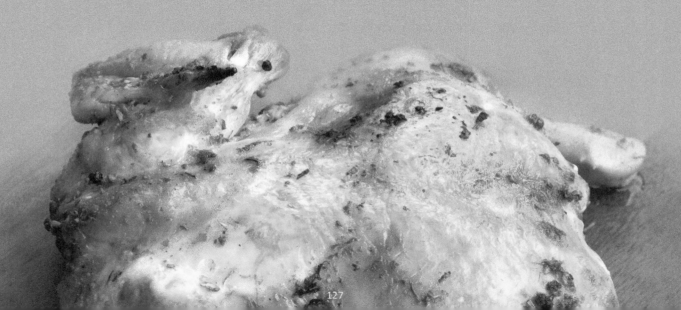

Zambian Chicken Stew

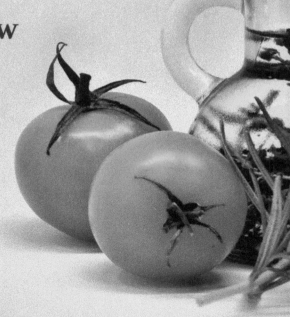

INGREDIENTS:

7 pieces of chicken, recommend chicken thighs

1 whole tomato

½ large Onion

½ Cup Vegetable Oil

½ Cups water

1 teaspoon Garlic Powder

1 teaspoon Seasoned Salt

1 teaspoon Onion Powder

1 teaspoon Chicken Spice

1 teaspoon Chicken Broth (powder)

½ teaspoon Curry Powder

PREPARATIONS:

1. In a medium pot, add the chicken and the water. Let the chicken boil on medium heat for about 30 minutes. Remove from stove and let it cool.

2. Remove the chicken from the pot but don't throw out the broth, we will need it later.

3. Heat oil in a pan (I would suggest a non- stick pan). Once oil is heated, add the chicken and fry on both sides until golden brown. When the chicken is all fried, remove some of the oil from the pan and leave enough for the gravy.

4. Then use the same pan to fry the onions and the tomatoes. Once those are cooked, add the gravy to the broth that you set aside. Then start adding the seasonings. Once the seasonings are mixed in with the gravy, add the fried chicken to the gravy and let it simmer on medium low for about 30 minutes or so. The chicken will be ready once the gravy is thick. Enjoy!

Recipe Notes

Recipe Notes

"

"I'm very consistent about spending time with
family. And when you have dinner with your
daughters - they'll keep you in your place and
they'll teach you something about perspective."

- Barack Obama

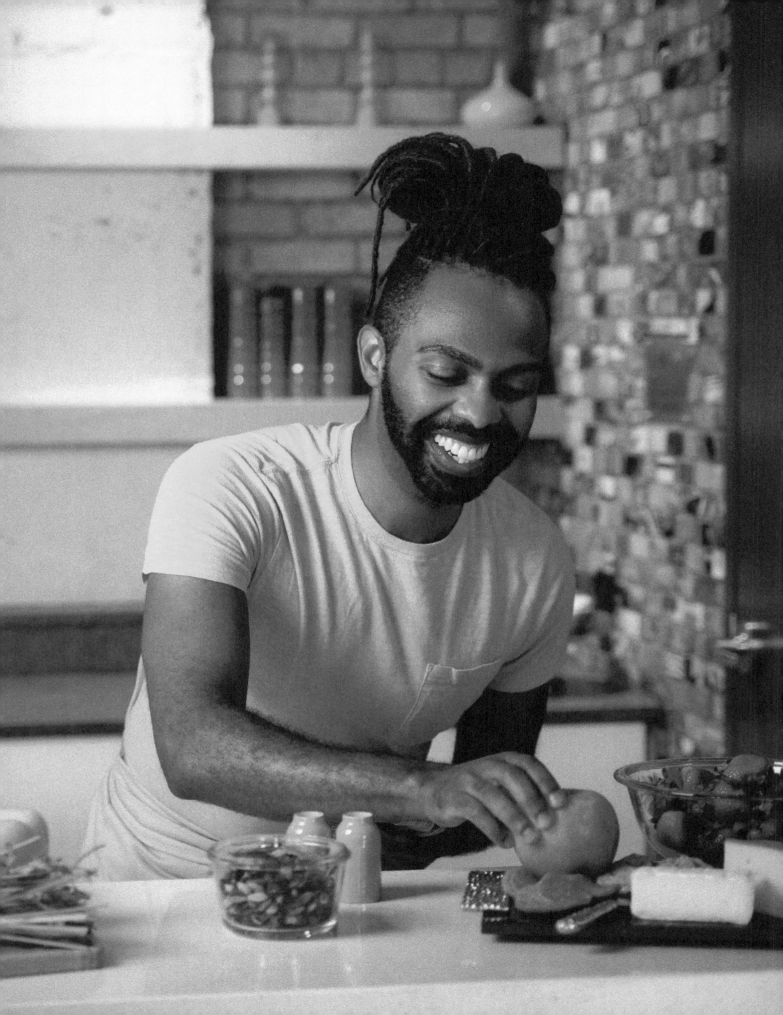

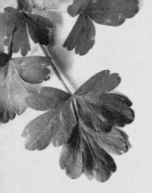
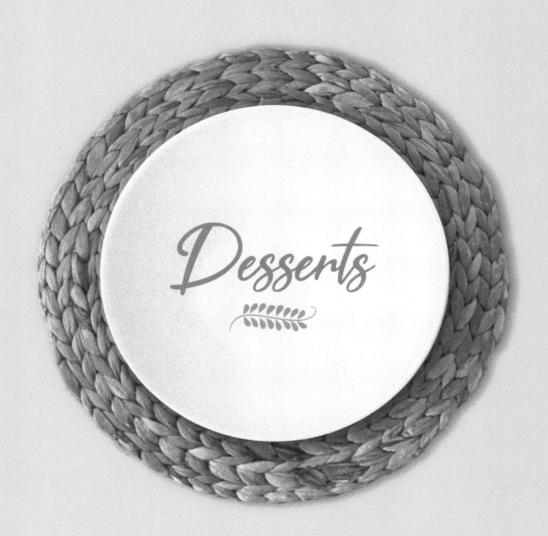

Desserts

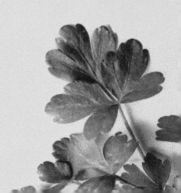

Carrot Souffle

INGREDIENTS:

2 cups cooked, pureed carrots

2 tsp lemon juice

2 Tblsp minced onion

½ cup butter, softened

¼ cup sugar

1 Tblsp flour

1 tsp salt

¼ tsp cinnamon

1 cup whole milk

3 eggs, room temperature

2qt Soufflé dish

PREPARATIONS:

1. Preheat oven to 350°F.
2. Beat all ingredients until smooth, and pour into a lightly buttered 2 quart soufflé dish.
3. Bake uncovered 45 minutes to 1 hour.

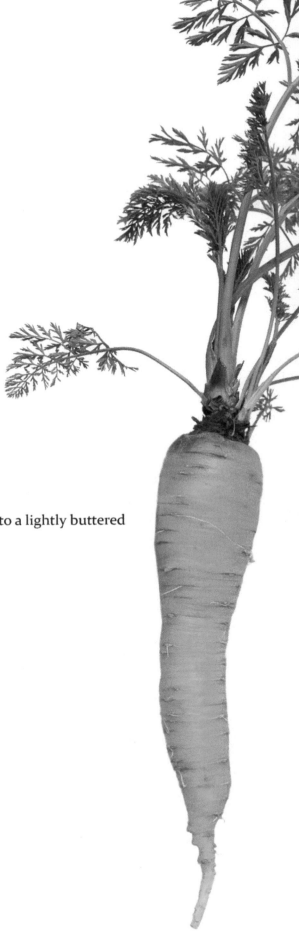

Grandma Nellie's Jubilee Jumbles

Also known as White Chocolate Chip Cookies!

INGREDIENTS:

1/2 cup shortening

1 cup brown sugar

1/2 cup white sugar

2 eggs

1 cup carnation evaporating milk

1 teaspoon vanilla extract

2 3/4 cup flour

1/2 teaspoon soda

1 teaspoon salt

PREPARATIONS:

1. Blend the shortening, brown sugar, white sugar, eggs, carnation milk, and vanilla extract.
2. Then add the flour, soda, and salt.
3. Mix the chocolate chips in, and let chill for 1 hour before baking.
4. Preheat the oven to 375 degrees. Line a large baking sheet with parchment paper or spray with nonstick cooking spray.
5. Scoop one heaping Tablespoon of dough at a time into a ball and place on the prepared pan about 1 - 1 1/2 inches apart. Bake cookies in preheated oven for 10-12 minutes, or until slightly golden around the edges.
6. Allow cookies to cool for 5 minutes before removing from pan.

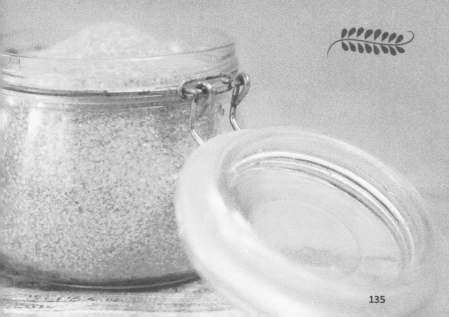

Ginger Snap Cookies

INGREDIENTS:

3/4 shortening

1 cup white sugar

1/4 cup light molasses

1 beaten egg

2 cup flour

1/4 teaspoon salt

2 teaspoons soda

1 teaspoon cinnamon

1 teaspoon clove

1 teaspoon ginger

PREPARATIONS:

1. Preheat the oven to 375° degrees
2. Blend together the shortening, white sugar, light molasses, and egg.
3. Then add the flour salt, soda, cinnamon, clove, and ginger.
4. Roll into small balls and then roll in sugar.
5. Bake at 375° degrees for about 15 minutes.

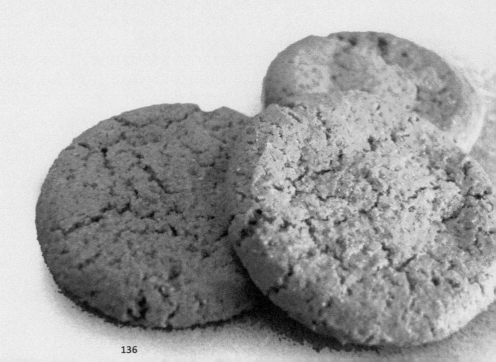

Laurie's Carrot Cake

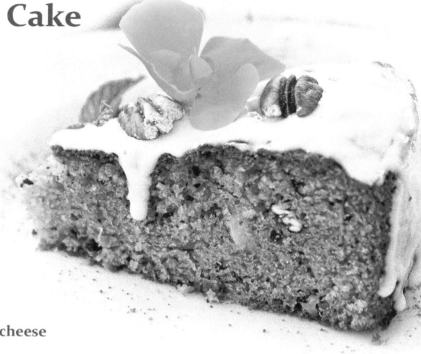

INGREDIENTS:

3 1/2 cups shredded carrots

2 cups sugar

1 1/4 cups vegetable oil

4 eggs

2 cups all purpose flour

2 teaspoons of baking soda

1/2 teaspoon salt

2 teaspoons cinnamon

FROSTING INGREDIENTS:

8 ounce package softened cream cheese

1/2 cup softened butter

2 1/2 cups powdered sugar

1 1/2 teaspoons vanilla

PREPARATIONS:

1. Heat oven to 350

2. Grease and flour 9 x 13 pan

3. In mixer combine carrots, sugar, oil, eggs. Add flour, soda, salt and cinnamon mixing until well blended. Pour into greased and floured 9 x 13 pan. Bake for about 30 minutes or until toothpick inserted in the center comes out clean.

4. For frosting combine all ingredients and mix until well blended. Spread on cooled cake.

Grandma Kelly's/Mimi's Apple Pie

INGREDIENTS:

8- 10 Green Apples or Haralson apples *peeled, cored and sliced*

1 teaspoon cinnamon

1/2 stick sliced butter

2 cups flour

1/2 cup lard

3/4 teaspoon salt

1 1/2 cups sugar

INGREDIENTS FOR CRUST:

2 cups flour

1/2 cup lard

3/4 teaspoon salt

1 1/2 cups sugar

INGREDIENTS FOR FILLING:

8- 10 Green Apples or Haralson apples *peeled, cored and sliced*

1 teaspoon cinnamon

1/2 stick sliced butter

PREPARATIONS

1. Mix flour, salt and sugar. Cut lard into mixture. Mix until the ingredients hold together. Knead and form dough into two balls, dust with flour and wrap in plastic and refrigerate for one hour. Take out and let stand for a few minutes. Place each ball on a floured surface and roll into 12" circle.

2. Place bottom crust into glass pie pan letting the edge fall over the sides. Fill with apples, cinnamon and butter. Add top crust and press the edges together. Make slits in the top of the pie crust.

3. Bake at 425° for 35 - 40 minutes

Mimi's Chocolate Brownies

INGREDIENTS:

1 1/2 cups sugar

2/3 cup melted butter

4 eggs well beaten

1 cup flour

1/2 teaspoon baking powder

Pinch of salt

3 squares baking chocolate

1 can whole walnuts

1 teaspoon vanilla

PREPARATIONS:

1. Bake in 350 degree oven

2. 8 inch square pan (Double recipe for a 9 x 13 pan) Mix in order given. Bake 1 hour until toothpick comes clean.

3. Frost with favorite chocolate frosting recipe or use Betty Crocker chocolate frosting.

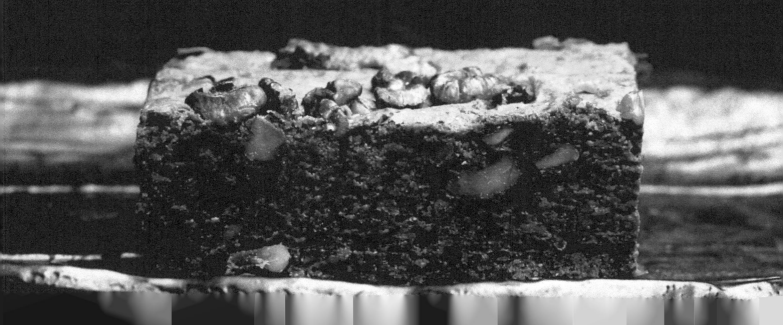

Mimi's Fudge

INGREDIENTS:

4 1/2 cups sugar

2- 7 ounce Hershey candy bars

1 can carnation evaporated milk

1 teaspoon vanilla

1/4 cup butter

1-12 ounce bag chocolate chips

1 can walnuts

16 large marshmallows

PREPARATIONS:

1. Use a 9 x 13 pan
2. Combine sugar, milk, and butter in saucepan. Bring to rolling boil for 5 minutes stirring constantly. Add Hershey bars, chocolate chips and marshmallows. Add nuts and vanilla.
3. Pour into buttered 9 x 13 pan.

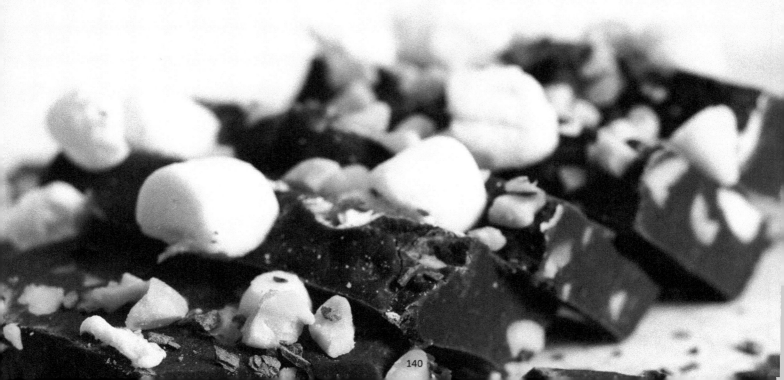

Pumpkin Chiffon Pie

CRUST INGREDIENTS:
1 graham cracker crumb crust
1 cup graham cracker crumbs
½ cup chopped walnuts
2 Tbsp sugar
¼ cup melted butter

PIE FILLING INGREDIENTS:
¾ cup brown sugar
1 envelope unflavored gelatin
½ tsp salt
1 tsp cinnamon
½ tsp nutmeg
¼ tsp ginger
3 lightly beaten egg yolks
¾ cup whole milk
1 ¼ cup canned pure pumpkin
3 egg whites
1/3 cup granulated sugar

CRUST PREPARATIONS:
1. Mix all ingredients together. Press into bottom and sides of pie pan.
2. Bake at 400F for 7 minutes (until lightly browned). Chill in refrigerator.
3. [Best if prepared the day before the filling and kept chilled]

PIE FILLING PREPARATIONS:
1. In saucepan, combine brown sugar, gelatin, salt and spices. Combine egg yolk and milk; stir into dry ingredients in the saucepan. Cook over low to medium heat, stirring constantly, until mixture boils. Remove from heat and stir in pumpkin. Chill in refrigerator until mixture mounds slightly when spooned (~ ½ hour).
2. Beat egg whites until soft peaks form. Gradually add granulated sugar and beat until stiff peaks form. Fold egg whites into pumpkin mixture. Turn into cooled, baked graham cracker crumb crust. Chill.

Recipe Notes

Recipe Notes

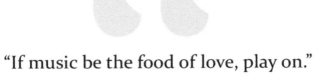

"If music be the food of love, play on."

- William Shakespeare

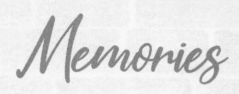

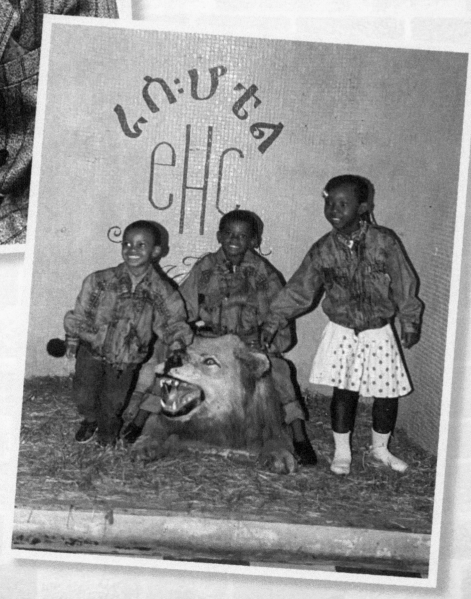

Memories

Storytime

Edena

We had a new stereo system in the living room that my husband Robert had gotten. Edena and Kasano were in the living room by themselves, and Edena was poking around the stereo system. He started poking and playing with the plug-in that the stereo system was plugged into, and as a result it would spark. This of course excited Edena, so he continued to do so. The speaker must have had enough because there was a thud and it started to smoke. Edena decided to go and get blankets, pillows, and anything, including paper, that he could use to put on top of the speaker to hide it. The smoke started getting thicker and bigger. Before you know it the spark from the plug-in started a fire, and it rose to the sealing in one straight line in a matter of seconds. At this moment Kasano, who had been watching his big brother in disbelief, screamed and ran to get the adults. Edena, scared he would get in trouble, shut and locked the door, and put the key in his pocket.

We were in the kitchen having lunch, and Robert was at work. I just put a big cake in the fridge because the next day was Mpango's birthday. Kasano came bursting into the kitchen screaming and saying we need to come to the living room. We all ran over and the smell was so strong, you could tell it was a fire. We started banging on the door and saying "Open the door! Edena! Open the door!", but he was scared!

He finally opens the door and the smoke billowed out of the living room. We grabbed Edena and his hair was white! We immediately started getting important things out of the house, it was an electrical fire and the ceiling was high. The fire was getting worse!

In Zambia fire trucks bring water with them, and we could finally hear that it arrived...but to our dismay, the fire truck didn't have any water...they ran out. So everyone in the neighborhood grabbed buckets and started throwing water from their own sinks at the house, but the fire was up high and it was an electrical one. We could do nothing but watch the whole house burn to the ground. We obviously moved that night.

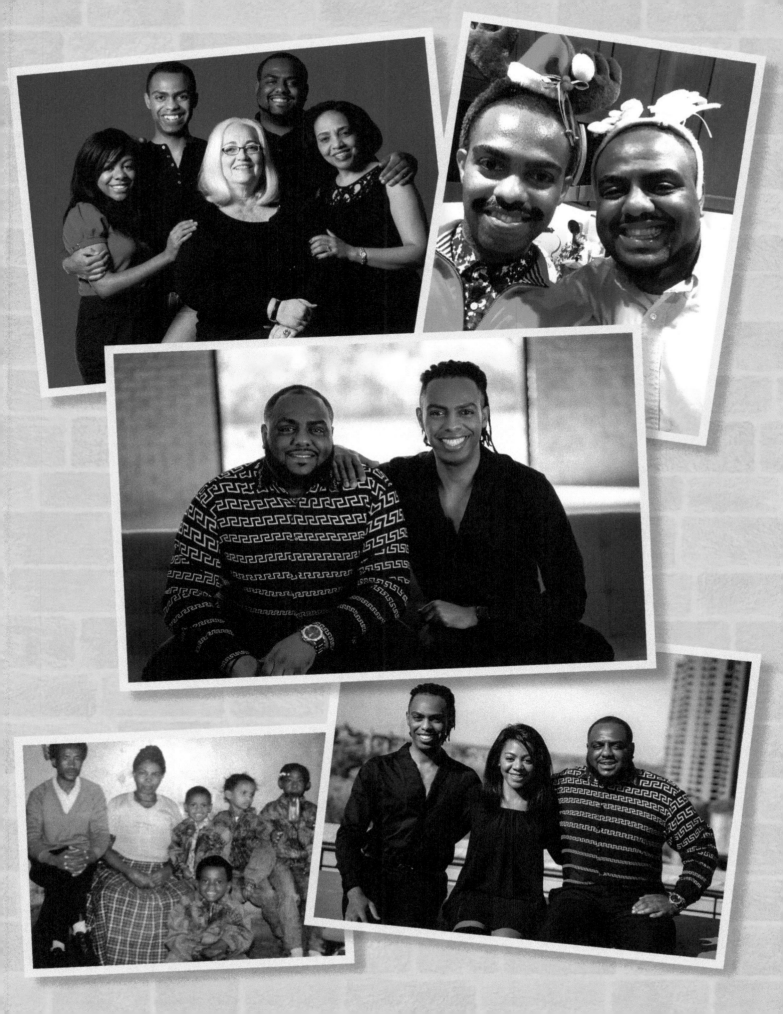

In Loving Memory

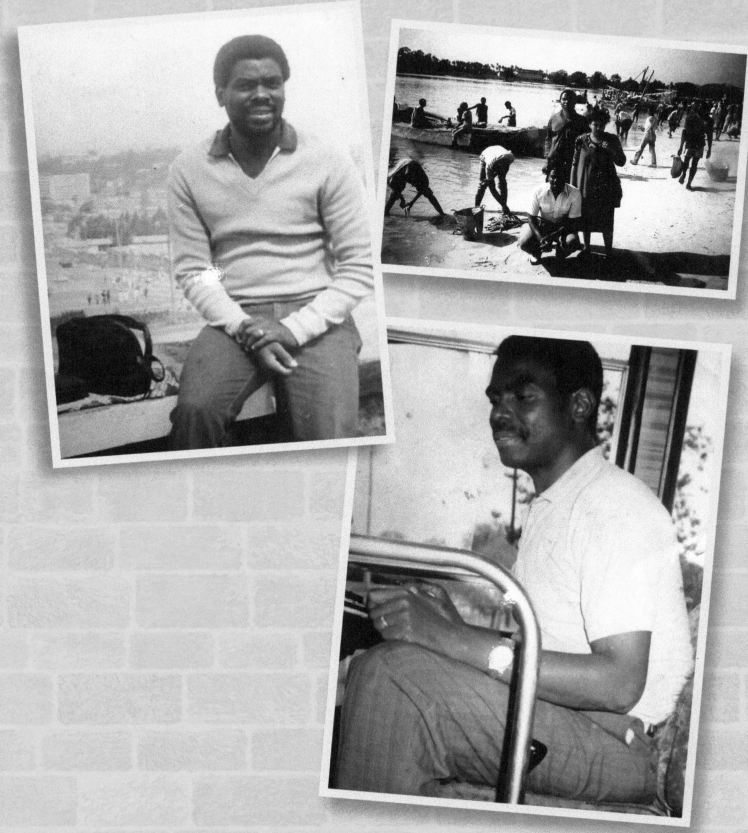

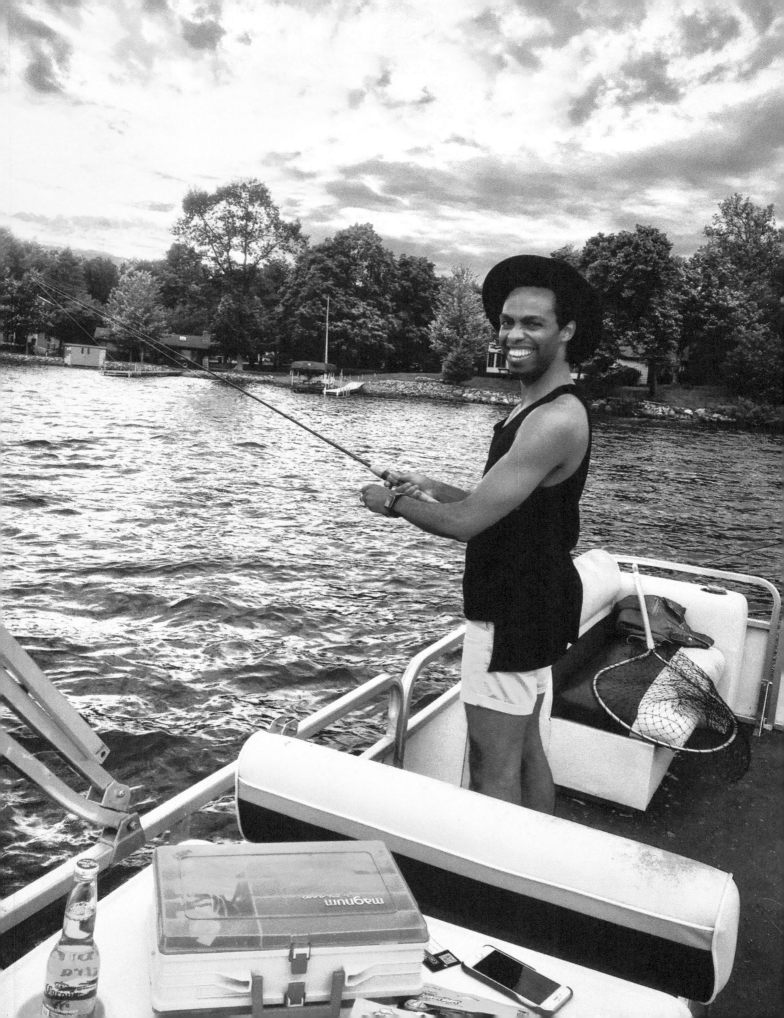

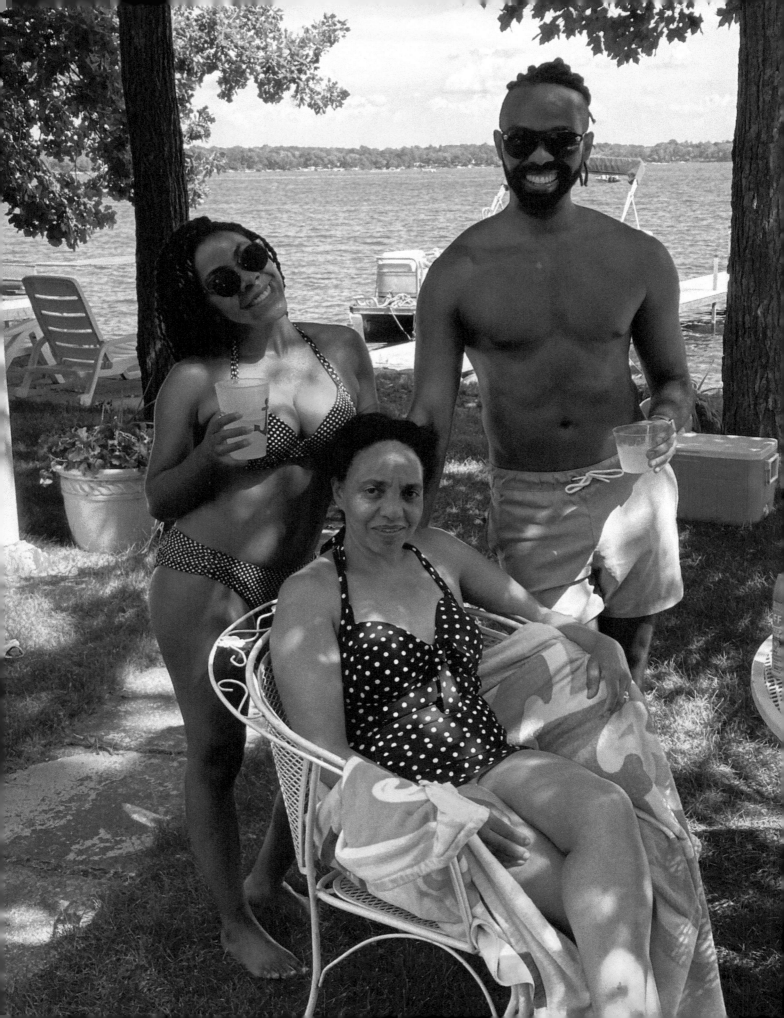

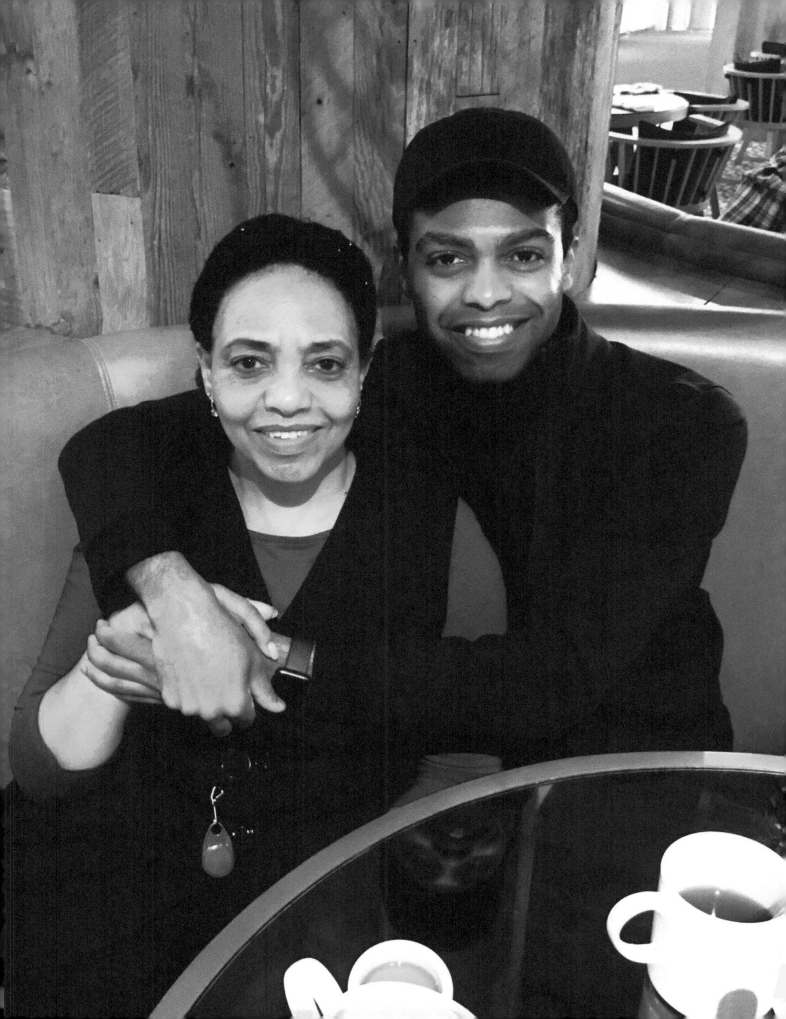

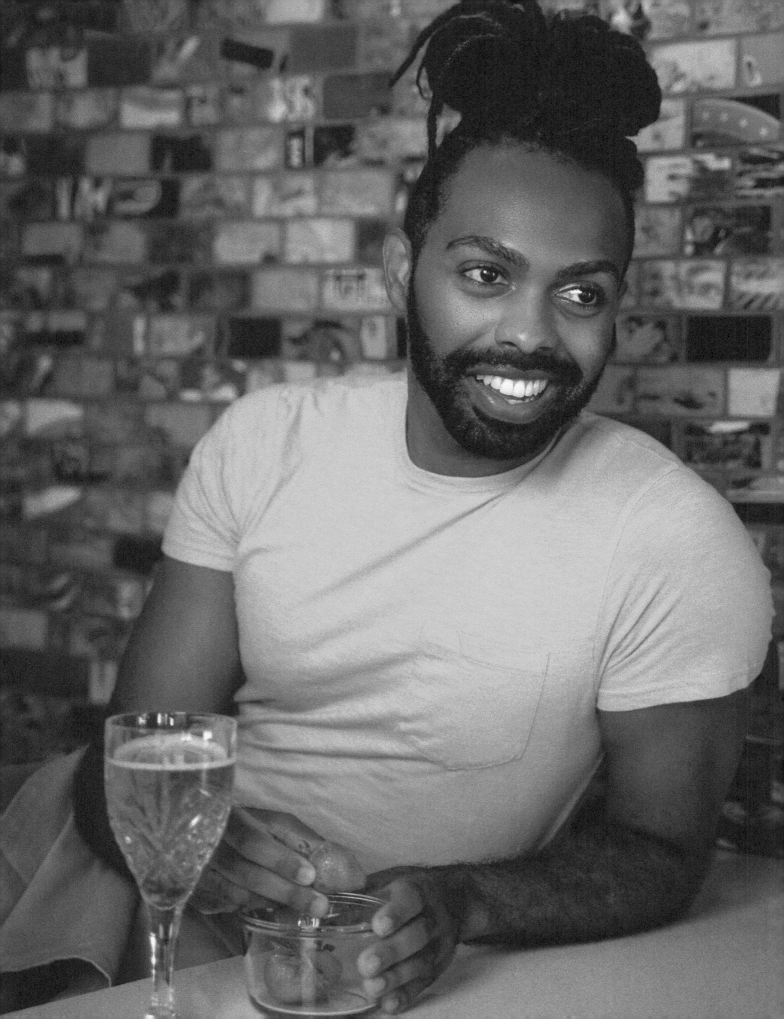

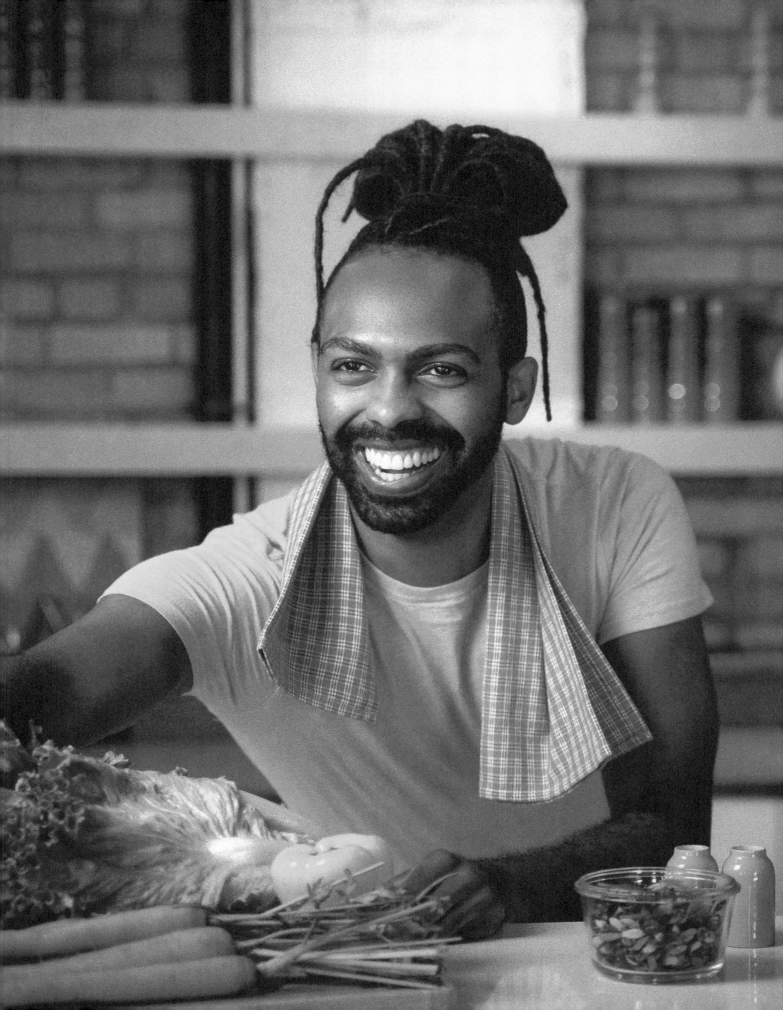

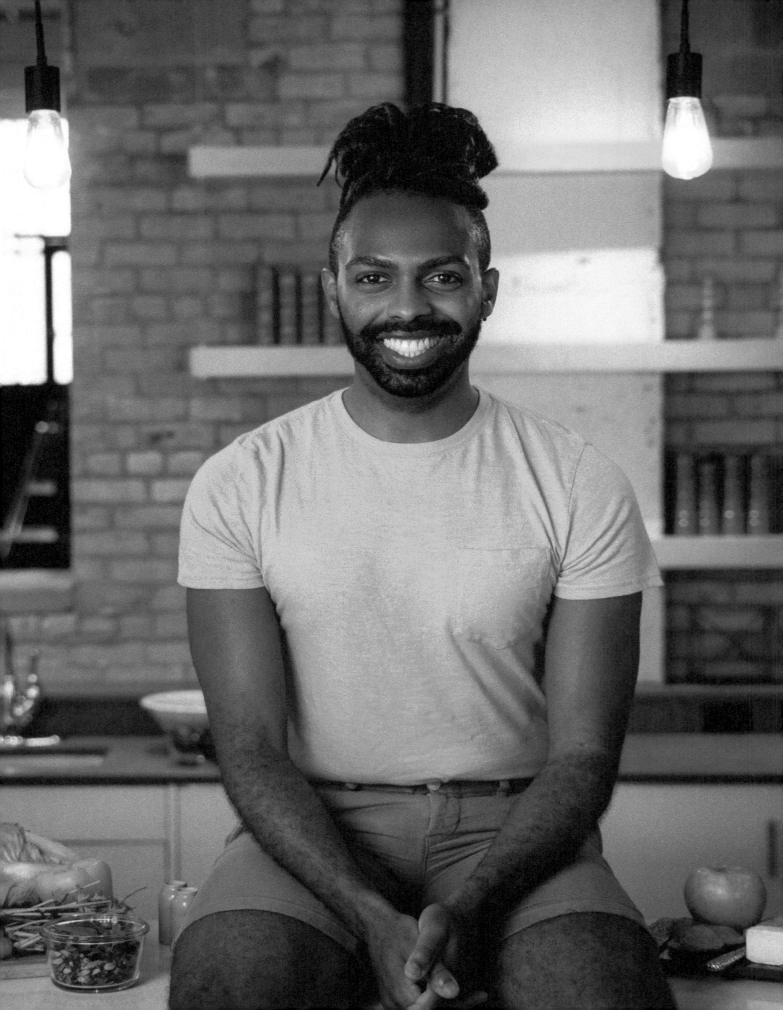

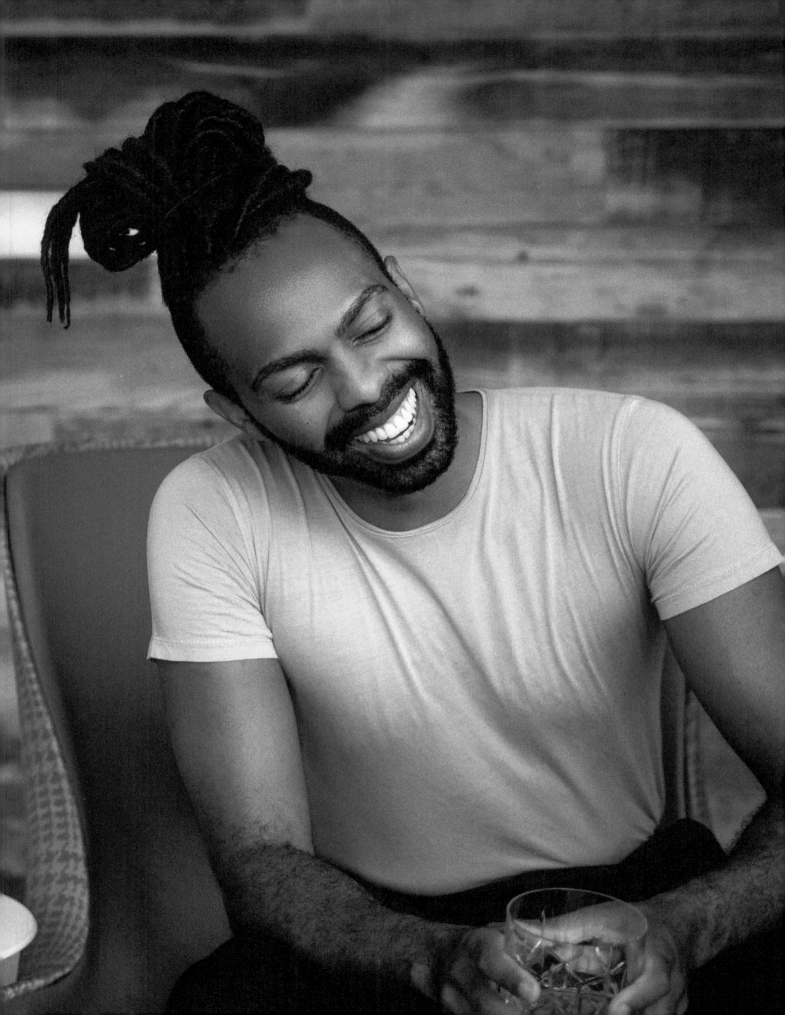

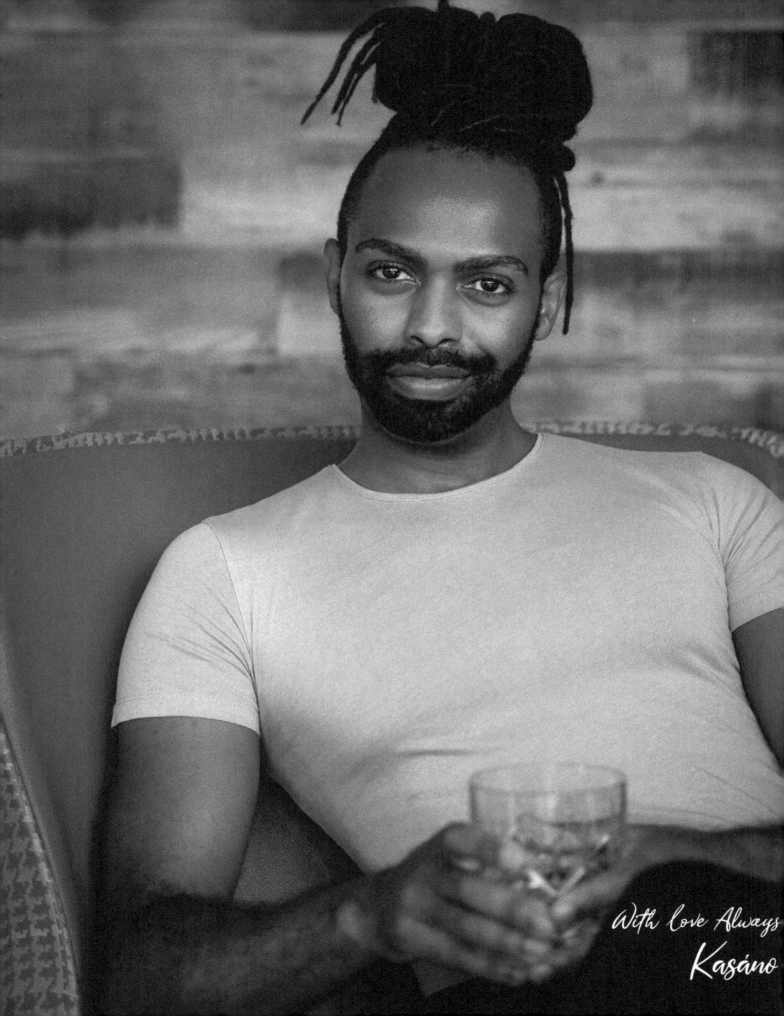

With love Always
Kasáno

Recipe Notes

Recipe Notes

Recipe Notes

Recipe Notes

Recipe Notes

Recipe Notes

Recipe Index

CPSIA information can be obtained
at www.ICGtesting.com
Printed in the USA
LVHW071701050121
675552LV00023B/786